Histology
Text and
PowerPoint Presentation

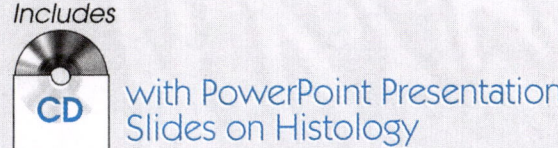

Includes

CD with PowerPoint Presentation
Slides on Histology

Histology

Text and
PowerPoint Presentation

Chief Editor

S Saritha MBBS, MS (Anatomy)

Professor and Head
Department of Anatomy
Kamineni Academy of Medical Sciences and
Research Center, Hyderabad

Editor

K Kshitija MBBS, MD (Pathology)

Assistant Professor
Department of Pathology
Apollo Institute of Medical Sciences and
Research Center, Hyderabad

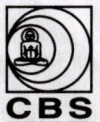

CBS

CBS Publishers & Distributors Pvt Ltd

New Delhi • Bengaluru • Chennai • Kochi • Kolkata • Mumbai
Hyderabad • Jharkhand • Nagpur • Patna • Pune • Uttarakhand

Histology
Text and
PowerPoint Presentation

ISBN: 978-93-87085-88-6
First Edition: 2018
Copyright © Chief Editor and Publisher

Published by Satish Kumar Jain and produced by Varun Jain for

CBS Publishers & Distributors Pvt Ltd
4819/XI Prahlad Street, 24 Ansari Road, Daryaganj, New Delhi 110 002, India.
Ph: 23289259, 23266861, 23266867   Website: www.cbspd.com
Fax: 011-23243014   e-mail: delhi@cbspd.com; cbspubs@airtelmail.in.
Corporate Office: 204 FIE, Industrial Area, Patparganj, Delhi 110 092
Ph: 4934 4934   Fax: 4934 4935   e-mail: publishing@cbspd.com; publicity@cbspd.com

Branches

* **Bengaluru:** Seema House 2975, 17th Cross, K.R. Road, Banasankari 2nd Stage, Bengaluru 560 070, Karnataka
  Ph: +91-80-26771678/79   Fax: +91-80-26771680   e-mail: bangalore@cbspd.com
* **Chennai:** 7, Subbaraya Street, Shenoy Nagar, Chennai 600 030, Tamil Nadu
  Ph: +91-44-26680620, 26681266   Fax: +91-44-42032115   e-mail: chennai@cbspd.com
* **Kochi:** Ashana House, No. 39/1904, AM Thomas Road, Valanjambalam, Ernakulam 682 016, Kochi, Kerala
  Ph: +91-484-4059061-65   Fax: +91-484-4059065   e-mail: kochi@cbspd.com
* **Kolkata:** 6/B, Ground Floor, Rameswar Shaw Road, Kolkata-700 014, West Bengal
  Ph: +91-33-22891126, 22891127, 22891128   e-mail: kolkata@cbspd.com
* **Mumbai:** 83-C, Dr E Moses Road, Worli, Mumbai-400018, Maharashtra
  Ph: +91-22-24902340/41   Fax: +91-22-24902342   e-mail: mumbai@cbspd.com

Representatives

• Hyderabad	0-9885175004	• Jharkhand	0-9811541605	• Nagpur	0-9021734563
• Patna	0-9334159340	• Pune	0-9623451994	• Uttarakhand	0-9716462459

Printed at: Mudrak, Patparganj, Delhi, India

Preface

I am pleased to introduce this new concept publication *Histology* in the form of PowerPoint slides accompanied by relevant text material on the topics described in the PPt slides. These slides are simplified with scientific material in histology.

I have made efforts to give rich, clear and precise orientation and interpretation in each section with animation, wherever possible, for understanding of the undergraduate and postgraduate medical students as well as the teaching faculty.

This endeavor would have been lost in the ocean but for her husband, Dr Kumarswamy, for his constant inspiration and endurance.

I express my deep sense of gratitude to my teachers for their blessings. I also express my deep love to my daughter Dr K Kshitija and her junior staff Dr T V Ramani for constant support in preparing the PowerPoint slides and the related text material.

I will regard as a reward if the PowerPoint presentation on histology receives constructive criticism for improvement.

S Saritha
Chief Editor

Contents

General Histology

1. Epithelial Tissue
2. Connective Tissue
3. Cartilage
4. Bone of Osseous Tissue
5. Muscle
6. Nerve
7. Circulatory System
8. Lymphoid System (Immune System)
9. Skin and its Appendages (Integumentary System)

1

Epithelial Tissue

Cells that work together in functionally related groups called tissues.

Types of tissues: These are four basic tissues in the body

1. Epithelial—lining and covering
2. Connective—support
3. Muscle—movement
4. Nervous—control

Four primary tissues of the body—developmentally

1. Epithelial tissue—ectoderm or mesoderm or endoderm
2. Connective tissue—mesoderm
3. Muscle tissue—mesoderm or ectoderm
4. Nervous tissue—ectoderm

Location of epithelial tissue

1. Sheets of cells that covers external surfaces of the body (skin).
2. Lines (internal) luminal surfaces of the cavities (esophagus, trachea).

Functions

1. Selective barrier
2. Protection of tissues
3. Closed cavities

4. Urothelium
5. Sensory functions.

Characteristics
1. Predominantly cellular
2. Mitotic activity
3. Avascular (except internal ear)
4. Special proteins
5. Rests on the basement membrane.

Basement membrane
Noncellular supporting sheet between epithelium and connective tissue.

Functions
Acts as a selective filter, determining which molecules from capillaries enter the epithelium. Acts as regenerating of epithelial cells.

It has two layers: Basal lamina and reticular layers. The underlying connective tissue or superficial fascia is deep to it.

Classification of Epithelial Tissue Cell Layers and Morphology of Surface Cells: Three Types
1. Simple epithelium or unilaminar: Single layer of cells.
2. Multilayered epithelium or stratified epithelium: It consists of many layers of cells.
3. Highly specialized tissue: It consists of heterogeneous population of cells forming lineage of spermatozoa EG. Seminiferous epithelium of the testis.

Classification of epithelial tissue indicates number of layers
 I. Simple epithelium consists of one layer of cells
II. Stratified epithelium consists of more than one layer of cells.

I. SIMPLE EPITHELIUM ACCORDING TO SHAPE

There are four types:

1. Squamous epithelium: Flat cells, height very little than width.
2. Cuboidal epithelium: Height and width of the cells are more less equal.
3. Columnar epithelium: Height of cells greater than width.
4. Pseudostratified ciliated columnar epithelium: All cell bases touch the basement membrane, not the lumen and nuclei are at different levels.

Cell shape depends upon cell volume and metabolic activity

i. Low metabolic activity—little cytoplasm with a few organelles, e.g. squamous and cuboidal cells
ii. High metabolic with abundant mitochondria—ciliated and secretary, e.g. tall columnar cells.

1. Simple Squamous Epithelium or Pavement Epithelium

Cytoplasm forms thin layer and nucleus bulges of the surface

Examples

1. Mesothelium—serous cavities
2. Endothelium—blood vessels and lumphatics
3. Heart—endocardium
4. Lungs—simple squamous epithelium.

Function correlation of simple squamous epithelium

Passage of materials by passive diffusion and filtration (gases in lungs and fluids across blood capillaries).

Secretes thin tissue fluid into the cavities for lubricating and preventing friction in serosa.

Location

Renal corpuscles, alveoli of lungs, lining of heart, blood and lymphatic vessels.

Lining of ventral body cavity (serosa)

In peritoneal cavity simple epithelium reduces friction between visceral organs by producing lubricating fluids and transports fluid.

CVS: Endothelium allows for passive transport of fluids, nutrients and metabolites across the thin capillary walls to surrounding cells.

Lungs: Simple squamous epithelium provides gas exchange or transport between alveoli and capillaries.

2. Simple Cuboidal Epithelium: Height and Width are Same

Description: Single layer of cube-like cells with large, spherical central nuclei.

Function: Secretion, excretory and absorption.

Location: Kidney tubules, small excretory ducts of salivary glands and pancreas, germinal epithelium of ovary, thyroid follicles, proximal convoluted tubules and pigment layer of retina.

3. Simple Columnar Epithelium: Height is More than the Width

Description: Single layer of column-shaped (rectangular) cells with oval nuclei (basal, central or apical). Some bear cilia at their apical surface may contain goblet cells.

Function: Absorption, secretion of mucus and enzymes, and other substances.

Ciliated type propels mucus or reproductive cells by ciliary action.

Simple columnar epithelium modifications

1. Non-ciliated form
2. Ciliated form
3. Stereocilia

i. Non-ciliated form

Tall columnar cells with microvilli, e.g. striated border in small intestine.

Secretion and absorption: Lines digestive tract stomach → anus, gallbladder, ducts of some glands.

ii. Ciliated form

Tall columnar cells with cilia. Lines upper respiratory system (bronchi), uterine tubes, uterus and central canal of spinal cord. Moves fluids and particles along the passages.

iii. Stereocilia (nonmotile)

Tall columnar cells with large nonmotile branched microvilli, e.g. organ of Corti, vas deferens and epididymis. Main function is absorption.

Simple columnar epithelium: Function-secretary and absorption

Location, e.g.

1. Simple columnar—stomach
2. Ciliated columnar—upper respiratory tract, uterine tube
3. Simple columnar with microvilli
    a. Striated border—small intestine.
    b. Brush border—gallbladder.
4. Simple columnar—Stereocilia, vas deferens and organ of Corti.

4. Pseudostratified Columnar Epithelium

Description: All cells originate at basement membrane. Only tall cells reach the apical surface. May contain goblet cells and bear cilia.

Nuclei lie at varying heights within cells. Gives false impression of stratification.

Function: Secretion of mucus and propulsion of mucus by cilia.

Pseudostratified Columnar Epithelium—two types

1. Non-ciliated type: Ducts of male reproductive tubes and ducts of large glands.
2. Ciliated variety: Lines trachea and most of upper respiratory tract.

Functional correlation of simple cuboidal and simple columnar epithelium

1. Simple cuboidal epithelium line ducts of glands and organs. Covers the surface for protection.
2. In kidneys, the epithelium functions in transport, absorption of filtered substances and active secretion of substances from filtrate.
3. Simple columnar epithelium of stomach secretes mucus covers surface and protects from corrosive gastric secretions.

Functional correlation of epithelium with striated border (small intestine) and brush border (kidney-PCT)

1. In small intestine striated border functions as absorption of nutrients. It is enhanced by villi with microvilli increase the surface area for absorption.
2. Goblet cells secrete mucus and protect the epithelium
3. In kidney PCT has simple cuboidal epithelium with brush border (microvilli) → absorbs nutrients and filtrate the passes through tubules.

Functional correlation of epithelium with cilia or stereocilia

1. In respiratory passages (trachea and bronchi), pseudo-stratified contains both goblet cells and ciliated cells. Motile cilia on columnar cells cleanse the inspired air and transport mucus and trapped particles across the cell surface to the oral cavity.
2. In epididymis and vas deferens. Pseudostratified with stereocilia are nonmotile like microvilli absorb excessive testicular fluid produced by testis.

5. Pseudostratified Epithelium is Present in Special Senses as Sensory Epithelium or Neuroepithelium (special senses)

It is three types

1. Olfactory epithelium.
2. Gustatory epithelium.
3. Vestibulocochlear epithelium.

1. *Olfactory epithelium*: Seen posterior superior part—roof of nasal cavity.

   Olfactory epithelium—three types: **Receptor cells—bipolar (microvilli), supporting cells and basal cells**

2. Gustatory epithelium present in tongue (anteior 2/3rds)

   Gustatory epithelium—three types cells: Receptor cells (hairs), supporting cells and basal cells.

3A. Organ of Corti (auditory): Three types of cells—hair cells (receptor with stereocilia), phalangeal cells and rod cells.

3B. Vestibular apparatus: Two types
   Hair cells (receptor with stereocilia) and supporting cells.

6. Myoepithelial Cells (Ectoderm and Endoderm)

Contractile associated with glands.

II. STRATIFIED EPITHELIUM: TWO OR MORE LAYERS PROTECTION: THREE TYPES

1. Stratified squamous epithelium: Two types
   i. Keratinized
   ii. Non-keratinized epithelium.
2. Transitional epithelium or urothelium
3. Stratified cuboidal or columnar epithelium.

1. Stratified Squamous Epithelium

i. Stratified squamous nonkeratinized, e.g. esophagus mainly for protection of moist surfaces and withstand wear and tear.

Deep cells are columnar, middle cells are cuboidal, superficial cells are flat cells.

ii. Stratified squamous keratinized epithelium—most superficial cell are scale and dead cells.

For example, skin of palm of hand: Protection from abrasion, desication and bacterial invasion.

2. Transitional Epithelium or Urothelium

It is multilayered (4–6 cell), thickness deep cells are cuboidal, middle cells are polygonal or pear (binucleate), superficial cells are umbrella (octoploidy).

Transitional epithelium: For example, bladder when contracted or stretched without damage and forms protective osmotic barrier (between urine and tissues).

3. Stratified Cuboidal and Columnar Epithelium

i. Stratified cuboidal epithelium: Two layers of cuboidal cells, e.g. excretory duct in salivary gland.

Ducts play a metabolically active role in gland function.

ii. Stratified columnar epithelium very rare and seen in the junctional zone (oral cavity with oropharynx, or oropharynx with nasopharynx) and large ducts.

iii. Specialized tissue is seminiferous tubules of testis (stratified cuboidal epithelium). Linage series of spermatogonic cells:

1. Spermatogonia,
2. Primary spermatocyte,
3. Secondary spermatocyte,
4. Spermatids, and
5. Serotile cells.

Applied Aspects

1. Tumors of epithelium are benign or malignant.
2. Carcinoma from squamous epithelium is squamous cell carcinoma and from glands is adenoma.

Metastases occur via blood stream or lymphatics can produce secondaries in the skin.

Connective Tissue

Connective tissue is the most widely distributed tissue in our body. Predominately consists cells and intercellular matrix (secreted by the cell). It is diverse of the four tissue types with a wide variety of functions. Connective tissue binds, anchors and supports various cells, tissues and organs in the body.

Development

1. Connective tissue mainly: Mesodermal in origin.
2. Neurilemma of nerves and neuroglia cells → ectoderm in origin.
3. Connective tissue → head regions are neural crest cells in origin.

Functions

1. Provides structural and mechanical support to various organs of the body.
2. Facilities the transport of substances between cells and blood vessels (diffusion).
3. Defensive: All antigens and antibody reaction takes place in the connective tissue.
4. Important trophic and morphogenetic roles in organization and influencing growth and differentiation of the tissues.

Connective tissue consists of two basic elements: Cells and extracellular material called matrix.

Matrix consists

1. Connective tissue fibers
2. Ground substance
3. Tissue fluid

Cells of connective tissue are fixed and wandering

These are seven types: Macrophages, fibroblasts, mast cells, plasma cells, pigment cells, fat cells and undifferentiated cells.

1. **Fibroblasts:** Secrete both fibers and ground substance of the matrix.
   - Fibroblast cells are common type. Most numerous cell of connective tissue.
   - Fibroblast concerned with production of collagen, reticular, elastic fibers and extracellular ground substance (matrix). These are flat and fusiform shape cell, show branching processes, nucleus and cytoplasm. Inactive or resting cell → fibrocyte.

2. **Macrophages:** Macrophage or histocyte or clasmatocyte (scavenger cells) (mononuclear phagocyte system) fixed or free. These are phagocytes that develop from monocytes.

   Function: Phagocytic cell ingest foreign material or dead cells.

   Examples are:
   a. Blood monocytes
   b. Lungs—dust cells
   c. Spleen, bone marrow and lymph nodes—littoral cells
   d. Liver sinusoids—Kupffer cells
   e. Brain—microglia
   f. Skin—Langerhans cell of epidermis
   g. Bones are osteoclasts

3. **Plasma cells:** Antibody secreting cells that develops from B lymphocytes.

Degenerative product of B lymphocyte: Rare in connective tissue. Seen in inflammation.

A plasma cell has cartwheel nucleus, –ve Golgi image and with Russel bodies.

4. **Mast cells:** Mastocytes or histaminocytes are modified basophils. Present along blood vessels and capsule. These are defensive and produce histamine that help dilate small blood vessels in reaction to injury. Mastocytes has granules (membrane bound vesicles) which release histamine and heparin.

5. **Adipocyte (fat cells)** or lipocytes are in groups or singly (signet ring appearance). Fat cells that store triglycerides, support, protect and insulate.
   1. White adipocytes unilocular. Nucleus is eccentrically located.
   2. Brown adipocytes multilocular, polygonal in shape, have a considerable volume of cytoplasm and multiple lipid droplets of varying size. Their nuclei are round and centrally located. Present in hibernating animals and newborn.

   Importantance
   i. Adipose tissue is very vascular, high metabolic activity and acts endocrine organ is sole source of Leptin.
   ii. Regulates carbohydrate and lipid metabolism.
   iii. Influences hypothalamus by suppressing appetite and food intake.

6. **Pigment cells** are mainly for protection:
   i. In skin from effect of ultraviolet rays of sun.
   ii. The dark-colored pigment in the choroid absorbs light and limits reflections within the eye that could degrade vision.

FIBERS OF CONNECTIVE TISSUE

Fibers are three types:

1. **Collagen fibers** are large fibers made of the protein collagen and are most abundant fibers. Promote tissue flexibility.

Types of collagen fibres:

Type I: Classical tendons, ligaments and dermis.

Type II: Hyaline cartilage, vitreous body.

Type III: Reticular fibers.

Type IV: Basal lamina of basement membrane.

Around 20 types are seen.

2. **Elastic fibres** or yellow fibers, e.g. ligamentum flava and wall of large arteries.

   Intermediate fibers run single, thick and made of the protein elastin. Branching fibers that allow for stretch and recoil.

3. **Reticular fibers** (type III, collagen fibers): Small delicate, branched fibers have same chemical composition of collagen. Forms structural framework in spleen and lymph nodes.

Connective tissue: Ground substance, extrafibrillar matrix. It occupies the space between cells and fibers. Routine preparations, it is lost during the fixation and dehydration process, and only cells and fibers can be seen.

Ground substance is viscid gelatinous material and amorphous colloidal substance distant from the tissue fluid which holds varying amount of water.

Forms the non-fibrous element of matrix within which cells and fibers are embedded.

1. H_2O serves as medium for diffusion of gases and metabolic products between blood vessels and cells *vice verse*.

2. Ground substance efficient barrier to spread of pathogens from connective tissue to blood.

3. Hyaluronic acid: Complex combination of polysaccharides and proteins.

EXAMPLES OF CONNECTIVE TISSUE

1. Loose Areolar CT

a. Consists of all three types of fibers, several types of cells, and semi-fluid ground substance.

b. Found in subcutaneous layer and mucous membranes, and around blood vessels, nerves and organs

c. **Function:** Strength, support and elasticity.

2. Dense Connective Tissue

It divided in two types

a. *Dense regular connective tissue*: Great tensile strength and pull along single axis, e.g. tendons and ligaments.

   i. Contains more numerous and thicker fibers and a few cells than loose CT

   ii. Consists of bundles of collagen fibers and fibroblasts

   iii. Tendons, ligaments and aponeuroses

   iv. **Function:** Provide strong attachment between various structures.

b. *Dense irregular connective tissue*: Withstand stress and strain in all directions, e.g. submucosa of digestive tract, dermis of skin (reticular layer) and adventitia of blood vessel.

SPECIAL CONNECTIVE TISSUES

These are reticular, adipose and elastic tissues.

1. Reticular tissue, e.g. lymph node

   i. Consists of fine interlacing reticular fibers and reticular cells

   ii. Found in liver, spleen and lymph nodes

   iii. **Function:** It forms the framework (stroma) of organs and binds together smooth muscle tissue cells.

2. Adipose tissue: It consists of adipocytes; "signet ring" appearing fat cells. They store energy in the form of triglycerides (lipids).

   ii. Found in subcutaneous layer around the organs and in the yellow marrow of long bones.

   iii. **Function:** It supports, protects and insulates. It also serves as an energy reserve.

3. Elastic tissue

Large artery (aorta) in the tunica media.

Functions

Loose areolar tissue holds structures together and facilitates movement (skin).

Dense irregular connective tissue—it maintains shape, resist pull in different directions.

Dense regular connective tissue—great tensile strength and strong resistance along single axis (tendon and ligaments).

Dura mater provides support and strength. Adipose tissue provides nutrition and generates heat. Leptin regulates lipid metabolism.

Diseases of Connective Tissue

Concerned with mutation of genes

1. Collagen fibers are not formed in the bones. Leads to weakness and break easily, e.g. osteogenesis imperforta.
2. Collagen diseases—skin becomes abnormal extensible and joints lax, e.g. Ehlers-Danlos syndrome.
3. Mutation of genes result in abnormal fibrillin (main consistuent of CF and EF):
   i. Subluxation of lens (weakness of suspensory ligament)
   ii. Rupture of aorta (tunica media EF)
4. Marfan's syndrome—abnormally tall because of deficient fibrillin.

Cartilage

Special Connective Tissue

Skeletal tissues like cartilage and bone are essential connective tissues in the body. It consists of cells embedded in the matrix, which is permeated by the fibers (collagen and elastic). Matrix of skeleton tissues are solidified.

Cartilage and bone differ in physical properties, vascularization, growth and regeneration.

Structure of Cartilage

Cartilage is phylogenetically ancient tissue widespread as permanent or temporary skeleton. In fetal life, the human skeleton is mostly cartilaginous.

Adult cartilage persists: (1) Synovial joints, (2) larynx wall, (3) trachea, (4) bronchial tube and (5) epiglottis.

It also presents in (1) the rib cage, (2) the ear, (3) the nose and (4) the intervertebral disc.

Function

i. Cartilage is a stiff load bearing, yet flexible connective tissue with low metabolic rate, cable of withstanding considerable degree of pressure.
ii. It is not as hard and rigid as bone but is stiffer and less flexible than muscle.
iii. Cartilage has *no* blood vessels or nerves except in the perichondrium.

Three types of cartilage

(1) Hyaline cartilage, (2) white fibrocartilage and (3) elastic cartilage.

4th type is cellular cartilage: It is thin septa of matrix between cells stage of early embryonic cartilage (mammalian pinna).

Components of cartilage

1. Cells load bearing: Chondrocytes that produce a large amount of extracellular matrix.
2. Extracellular matrix: It absorbs stress and protects the chondrocytes, composed of collagen fibers, elastin fibers abundant ground substance rich in proteoglycan.
3. Perichondrium.

Cells of Cartilage

Chondroblasts: Young and active cells, small irregular and bear number of filopodia and basophilic. Divide mitotically and produce matrix.

Chondrocytes: Mature, large cells, lose ability to divide with abundant lipid vacuoles and trapped in lacunae maintain the cartilage matrix.

INTERCELLULAR MATRIX—WATER FILLED GROUND SUBSTANCE

Made up of chondroitin sulfate, collagen, elastic fibers and chondrocytes surrounded by a membrane: Perichondrium.

Ground substance is amorphous gel, H_2O, carbohydrates (PAS), glycoprotein and traces of lipid.

Cartilage is semirigid tissue

1. Matrix stores energy, imparts elasticity and rigidity to cartilage.
2. The strength of cartilage is due to collagen fibers and the resilience is due to the presence of chondroitin sulfate.
3. Chondrocytes occur within spaces in the matrix, called lacunae.

Collagen and elastic fibers

Type I—white fibrous C, perichondrium.

Type II—hyaline C, vitreous, corneal strome and nucleus pulpous.

Perichondrium is outer membrane, surrounds the cartilage (vascular)

1. Outer fibrous layer—irregular collagen fibers (I)
2. Inner cellular layer:
   a. Spindle-shaped fibroblast cells
   b. Deeper cell is chondrogenic layer. Secretes matrix and cells.

Nutrition to Cartilage

Cartilage is avascular (not wholly true)

Perichondrium is vascular.

Cartilage proper: Nutrients and metabolites diffuse along the concentration gradients across the intervening matrix.

Cartilage cells invaded by nutrient vessel, it becomes calcified.

Anti-angiogenic factor in the cartilage inhibits vascular invasion.

1. Hyaline Cartilage (most abundant type)

i. Glossy, bluish, homogenous and firm consistency and elasticity.

ii. Perichondrium has two layers. Outer is fibrous, inner is cellular. Consisting of chondroblasts which are flat near perichondrium, rounded or angular cells in the deeper tissue.

iii. *Cartilage proper:* Chondrocytes lie singly or groups. Cell nests or isogenous cell groups occupying lacunae. Offspring of one parent chondroblasts.

iv. Matrix is basophilic. It consists of territorial matrix/lacunar capsule which is metachromatic and inter-territorial matrix that is pale stain (between cell nest).

Territorial matrix, stains dark purple (H and E) with collagen type I.

Interritorial matrix is basophilic, rich in acid chondroitin sulphate.

Chondrion is an isogenous groups together with enclosing pericellular matrix.

v. Intercellular matrix—homogenous basophilic contains type II collagen fibers (acidophilic) which are masked by ground substance which as chondroitin sulphate (similar refractive index).

Hyaline cartilage: Found in embryonic skeleton, at the ends of long bones, costal, nasal, laryngeal cartilages, trachea, bronchi and most of articular cartilage.

Function: Flexible, provides support, allows movement at joints.

2. Yellow Elastic Cartilage: Opaque in Fresh State

External ear, epiglottis and auditory tube corniculate, cuneiform, apex of arytenoid (laryngeal cartilage).

1. Typical chondrocytes in lacunae (surrounded by type I collagen fibers)
2. Matrix pervaded by yellow elastic fibers
3. Regular, branch, network and anatomizing and interlacing fibers
4. Perichondrium presents with two layers and vascular.

Functions of Elastic Cartilage

i. Thread-like network of elastic fibers within the matrix gives support, maintains shape, allows flexibility.

ii. Most sites elastic fibers occur at vibrational functions, i.e. *laryngeal cartilage* helps in sound wave production and *external ear cartilage* transmission of sound waves.

3. White Fibrous Cartilage

Contains bundles of collagen in the matrix that are usually more visible under microscopy.

  i. Dense fasciculated white collagen fibers (type I) with
  ii. Fibroblasts and small inter-fascicular groups of chondrocytes in lacunae.
  iii. Cells ovoid, a few rows in interterritorial matrix bundles of collagen fibers with hardly any ground substance.
  iv. Perichondrium—absent.

Function of white fibrous cartilage

Found in the pubic symphysis, intervertebral discs, acetabular and glenoidal labrum and menisci of the knee.

Function is to support and absorb shocks provide tensile strength and resist repeated pressure and friction (IV disc).

Appear-like tendon where fibroblast change to chondrocytes in lacunae.

Bone of Osseous Tissue

Bone is the major structural and supportive connective tissue of the body.

Osseous tissue forms the rigid part of the skeletal system.

Functions

1. Bone serves as skeleton for attachment for tendon and muscles.
2. Bone protects soft tissue like brain, heart lungs and urogenital organs.
3. Store house for Ca, PO_4 and other minerals, 90% of Ca is stored in bone (regulated by calcitonin and parathormone hormones).
4. Functions of hemopoietic tissue.

Characteristics of bone

i. Bone can only grow appositionally. Bone cannot grow interstitially, from within by the division of bone cells because of the presence of rigid calcium salts within the matrix.
ii. Bone similar to cartilage consists of cells and extracellular matrix (type I collagen fibres.)
iii. Bone matrix is acidophilic and bone is highly vascular.
iv. It is hard, rigid resilience and is regenerative.

Classification of bone

1. Macroscopic (2) types: Compact and cancellous bones.

2. **Developmental (2) types:** Intramembraneous (dermal) and intracartilagenous bones.

3. **Microscopic (2) types:** Lamellar bone (secondary osteon) and alamellar bone(primary osteon).

Macroscopic bone

i. Compact bone, e.g. shaft of long bone. Outer hard cortex is dense ivory like.

   Compact bone provides strength

ii. Cancellous bone (trabecular or spongy), e.g. inner part of the shaft. It has a honeycomb appearance with cavities. Lattice work of bars and plates (marrow) flat bone-ribs.

Developmental Classification

Intramembranous ossification and endochondral ossification.

• But bone is the same regardless of the pathway
• Process of bone formation: Ossification
• Process of mineralization: Calcification

   i. Intramembranous ossification: Mesenchyme cells differentiate into → osteoblasts → osteocytes → bone formation.

   ii. Endochondral ossification: Mesenchyme cells → chondroblasts and chondrocytes → cartilaginous model → osteoblasts and osteocytes → bone formation.

Microscopic Classification

i. Woven bone is alamellar bone with primary osteon. It is immature or pathologic bone. With more osteocytes and higher rate of turn over and is randomly oriented. It is weaker and more flexible.

ii. Lamellar bone or secondary bone: Created by remodeling woven bone. It is more organized, stress oriented, stronger and less flexible than woven bone.

Components of bone are two types

  i. Cells

  ii. Matrix

Matrix is acidophilic. It has two parts: Organic and inorganic substances.

Organic substances

  i. Collagen fibres type I, arranged in layers

  ii. Ground substances contains gycosaminogylcans, proteoglycan and H_2O.

Glycoprotein (osteonectin and osteocalcin) which play important role in mineralization.

Osteoid (secreted by osteoblasts): Mixture of collagen fibers + organic ground substance before mineralization.

Inorganic substances: Predominantly calcium (Ca) and phosphorus (phosphate).

Calcium phosphate, Ca carbonate, magnesium carbonate, Mg chloride, fluoride, Na and potassium—small amount.

65% of dry wt—inorganic salts

35%—organic substance.

Living bone—20% H_2O, 80% Ca salts. Ca salt is not fixed. Interchange with blood and bone by hormones (calcitonin and parathormone).

Cells of the bone

These are five types

Osteoprogenitor cells, osteoblasts, osteocytes, osteoclasts, bone lining cells.

Two categories of bone cells

  i. Osteoclasts are in the first category. They resorb the bone.

  ii. The other category is the osteoblasts family.

    1. Osteoblasts that form bone

    2. Osteocytes maintain bone

    3. Bone lining cells that cover the surface of the bone and protect the bone.

1. Osteoprogenitor cells (stem)

  i. Osteogenic cells are derived, pluripotent cells (periosteum and endosteum)
 ii. Mesenchymal stromal cells which give rise to other bone cells.
iii. Osteoprogenitor cells, irregular and elongated shape, with pale cytoplasm and pale nucleus. Proliferate and differentiate into osteoblasts.
 iv. In fetus, these cells are numerous at sites where bone formation occurs.
  v. In adult osteoprogenitor cells are present on bone surfaces.
 vi. Found along the blood vessels entering the cartilage.

2. Osteoblasts—bone forming cells; derived from osteoprogenitor cells

  i. Larger, roughly cuboidal mononuclear cells 15–30 µm, found on surfaces of the growing bone.
 ii. Single nucleus, basophilic cytoplasm, plenty of processes which come in contact with similar process of neighboring cells.
iii. Alkaline phosphate on surface of osteoblasts, helps in laying down the organic matrix and helps in calcification. This enzyme is shed and reaches the blood circulation and detected in rapid bone formation. Osteoblasts trapped in lacunae forms osteocytes.

Formation of bone in unequal sites of adult bone is an abnormal osteoblastic activity

  i. Ectopic bone formation.
 ii. Sclerotic arterial walls.
iii. Calcified foci of lungs or connective tissue.
 iv. Benign tumors of osteoblasts—osteoma.
  v. Malignant tumors—osteosarcoma.

3. Osteocytes: Major Cell Type of Mature Bone

  i. Scattered within the matrix, interconnected by numerous cellular extensions forming complex cellular network.

  ii. Derived from osteoblasts trapped in matrix, i.e. in lacunae, but retain contacts with each other and with cells at the bone surface throughout life span.

  iii. Ellipsoid (25 µm), oval nucleus, cytoplasm is acidophilic.

  iv. Numerous fine processes emerge from the cell body—branch like tree.

  v. Tips in contact with processes of adjacent—osteocytes cells.

  vi. At bony surfaces with osteoblasts and bone forming cells maintain electrical and metabolic continuity.

Osteocytes: Life span—25 years

  i. Processes occupy canaliculi which contain extracellular fluid and continues with blood vessels in haversian canals. Transport nutrients and metabolites.

  ii. Living osteocytes are essential for maintenance of organic matrix (Ca) of bone.

  iii. Maintenance of integrity of lacunae and canaliculi and keeps the channels open for nutrition.

4. Osteoclasts formed from Fusion of Mononuclear Cells: Reabsorption and Remodeling—Life Span 16 Days

  i. Large cells—20–100 µm.

  ii. Multinucleated—15–20

  iii. Found in active bone removal surfaces, howship lacunae/reabsorption bays.

  iv. Cytoplasm—foam-like, vacuolated with lysosomes.

  v. Cell surfaces at the site of reabsorption—highly folded known as ruffled membrane.

  vi. Osteoclastic activity is stimulated by PTH suppressed by calcitonin.

  vii. Osteoporosis—abnormal reabsorption of bone due to defect in osteoclastic activity.

5. Bone Lining Cells

i. Flat epithelium-like cells on resting adult bone surfaces, i.e. periosteal or endosteal.
ii. Attached to each other and with osteocytes.
iii. Regulate the osteoprogenitor and osteoclastic activity.

Functions of Periosteum

i. It provides attachment—tendons, ligaments and muscles. Fibers of tendon continue into outer layer as Sharpey fibers.
ii. Periosteum—nutritive, blood vessels, nerves and lymphatics enter and leave.
iii. Fibrous layer—limiting membrane, prevents bone tissue from spilling out into neighbor tissues.

Microscopic Organization of the Bone

Macroscopically all living bone is white.

i. *Compact bone* limited to the cortices of the bone providing strength. It thickness or architecture vary in different bones which reflects on shape, position and functional roles.
ii. *Cancellous bone* is present in the interior of long bone and at expanded ends, giving additional strength to the cortices and support to the marrow cavity.

Proportions of compact and cancellous bone depend upon on general composition of matrix.

Two distant types

- Lamellar (secondary osteon) which is seen in adult bone. Both compact and in cancellous bone.
- Alamellar bone (primary osteon) or woven bone. Seen in the early embryonic development of bone.

COMPACT BONE

Bone in adult made up of layers of lamellae. Each lamella is thin plate of bone. Consisting of collagen fibers in layers

+organic (osteoid) and mineral salts deposited in gelatinous ground substance.

Lamellae are arranged in concentric cylindrical rings

Even a small piece of bone made up of several lamellae placed over one another. Between adjoining lamellae are small spaces known as lacunae within which are osteocytes

i. Each lacuna contains one osteocyte.
ii. Radiating from lacunae are fine canaliculi. Canaliculi from one lacuna communicate with a canaliculi of other lacuna and with haversian canal.
iii. Delicate cytoplasmic processes of osteocyte occupy the canaliculi.
iv. Canaliculi contain extracellular fluid derived from blood vessels in the haversian canal.

TRANSVERSE SECTION OF COMPACT BONE

i. Lamellae—3 µm thick (6–8 in number) concentric rings, surround haversian canal—50 µm in diameter at center (blood vessels, nerves).
ii. Haversian system (secondary osteon) is round or ellipsoid 100–400 µm in diameter.
iii. Lacunae, canaliculi with osteocytes and processes
iv. Between cement lines are interstitial lamellae (homogenous matrix).
v. Surface parallel to external circumferential lamellae.
vi. Marrow—internal circumferential lamellae between ECL and ICL are haversian system.

The haversian system is the fundamental functional unit of compact bone. HC branch and anastomosis and communicate-marrow cavity and with external surface via-Volkmann canals (blood vessels + nerves).

21 million osteons in adult skeleton.

Compact bone: Several such osteons.

Longitudinal Section of Compact Bone

i. Haversian canal-course longitudinal (tube like) parallel to long axis of bone.

ii. Lamellae: Lacunae with osteocytes and processes in canaliculi are parallel.

iii. Volkmann canals (perforating channels) join HC, marrow cavity and periosteum, penetrate the lamellae directly.

iv. Cementing line limits the osteon.

Trabeculae Bone or Cancellous Bone

i. Number of bony lamellae in form of rods and plates inter-lacing

Lamellar organization of trabeculae bone is in form of branching and anatomizing curved plates or rods encloses the marrow cavity.

ii. Lamellae are thickness—50 to 400 µm.

iii. Marrow cavity: Blood vessels and nerves, hemopoietic or adipose tissue. Marrow cavity lined by endosteum tissue.

iv. External covered by periosteum with osteoblasts beneath is thin compact bone.

v. Lamellae enclose osteocytes in lacunae with radiating processes in canaliculi. Osteocytes nutrition by diffusion from medullary vessels.

vi. Osteoclasts present along marrow cavity.

vii. Thick trabeculae contain small osteons.

Woven bone: Primary osteon

Newly formed bone with no lamellar structure. Collagen fibers in bundles run randomly in different directions giving a woven appearance. It has more osteocytes per unit of volume and higher rate of turnover. It is weaker and more flexible.

Intramembranous Ossification

For example, skull bones are woven bone → trabeculae with hemopoietic tissue (diploe). At birth, membranous at angle-fontanella.

Endochondral Ossification

Bone develops in hyaline cartilage model.
1. Zone of reserve cartilage: Small and irregular cell
2. Zone of proliferation: Cells large, mitosis in parallel
3. Zone of hypertrophy
4. Zone of calcification
   Matrix is calcified
5. Zone of resorption
6. Spicule of cartilage and bone

Applied Histology

i. Maintenance of Ca levels, phosphorus, vitamin A, C and D is by diet.
ii. Deficiency of calcium reduces the mineral content of bone: Osteoporosis.
iii. Vitamin D also influences Ca levels on intestinal absorption.
iv. Deficiency in adult—osteomalcia
v. Deficiency in children—rickets.

Muscle

I. MICROSCOPIC STRUCTURE OF MUSCLE

Muscle tissue is specialized to posses wide range of movements.

Most important sign of life is movement. Muscle is derived from the Latin *musculus* meaning 'little mouse' because of the shape of muscles or when contracting look like mice moving under the skin.

Action

1. Move the limbs—locomotion.
2. Inflation the lungs.
3. Pump the blood from the heart.
4. Open and close the tubes (GIT).
5. Phagocytosis.
6. Cell division (mitosis).
7. Extension of processes—withdrawal painful stimuli.

All muscles development from mesoderm expect arrector pilorum of the skin and muscles of the eyeball, i.e. sphincter pupillae, dilator pupillae and ciliaris muscle from ectoderm.

Coverings of Muscle

i. Each muscle fiber delicates areolar tissue—endomysium. Number of muscle fibers form muscle fasciculus.
ii. Each muscle fasciculus-surrounded by dense connective—perimysium.

iii. Number of muscle fasciculi ensheathed by epimysium (connective tissue membrane) protective, allows blood vessels and nerves.

Muscles tissue is composed predominantly cells; myocytes.

Myocytes are elongated in one direction, referred as muscles fibers.

Types of muscles

These are three types

1. Skeleton muscle or striated or voluntary muscle.
2. Cardiac muscle (heart)
3. Smooth muscle or unstriated or involuntary muscle.

1. Skeleton Muscle or Striated (LM) or Voluntary Muscle (Transverse Striations)

1. Attached to bony skeleton.
2. Contract at will. Except muscles of breathing, swallowing, perineum and middle ear.
3. Somatic nerves.
4. Development: Somites and neural crest cells.
5. Bulk of muscle.
6. Powerful contractions—100 watt/kg.

2. Cardiac Muscle is Myocardium of Heart Extend to Walls of Large Veins

1. Cardiac myocytes—network linked electrically and mechanically as a unit.
2. Involuntary—ANS.
3. Transverse striations (faint)
4. Myocardial mantle—intraembryonic mesoderm.
5. Contractions are rhythmically, less powerful and resistant fatigue (3–5 watts/kg).

3. Smooth Muscle or Unstriated or Involuntary Muscle

1. Walls of viscera (hollow tubes)—GIT, RS, UGT, tunica media of artery, arrector pili and iris muscles and dartos (scrotum).

2. Absence of transverse striations.
3. Involuntary—ANS and hormonal.
4. Splanchnic pleuric mesoderm.

Transverse Section of Skeletal Muscle

Myofibrils arranged in groups: Field of Conheim.

Long cylindrical parallel bundles. Length 1–30 cm, diameter 10–100 μm.

Each muscle fiber is a syncytium. Fibres do not branch or anastomose.

Nuclei beneath-sacrolemma (multinucleated) (fusion numerous myoblasts).

Sarcoplasm shows alternate dark and light segments (Transverse striations (Λ and I bands)

1. Distinct cross striations: H and E stains.
2. Due to definite organization of myofilaments (actin and myosin)
3. Dark bands—A or Q (basophilic) anisotropic
4. Light bands—I or J (acidophilic) isotropic
5. A-band—rotates the plane of polarizing microscope strongly. Do not refract light equally in different planes.
6. I band rotates the plane of polarizing microscope lightly. Refract light equally in different planes.
7. A-band (A or Q) bisected by H-light line (Hensen line). Running in centre of H-line is M-line.
8. I-band (I or J) bisected by thin dark line Z-disc.
9. Sarcomere area between two consecutive Z-disc (contractile unit of striated muscle).
10. Each muscle fiber consists of number of myofibrils. Each myofibril made up fine myofilaments. Two types of myofilaments—actin and myosin.
11. Supplied—somatic nerves.
12. Powerful contractions—100 watts/kg. Tonicity and contractions depends upon nerve supply.

13. Multinucleated and peripheral beneath sacroplasm.
14. Elongated, cylindrical fibres run in bundles parallel and do not branch, anastomose. 1 mm 30 cm, diameter 10–50 µm.

II. CARDIAC MUSCLE IS MYOCARDIUM OF HEART

Continuous with Large Veins

Embryologically cardiac mesoderm—myocardial mantle
1. Cardiac muscle is structural-like skeletal muscle and functional like smooth muscle. Transverse striations +
2. Length—100 µm, diameter—10–15 µm. Chain of myocytes—synctium.
3. Myocytes, with single centrally placed nucleus. Perinuclear zone: Halo where no myofibrils.
4. Cardiac myocytes branch and anastomose. Like a quadrangular fork.
5. Transverse striations are similar to skeleton muscle but faint (A, I, Z, H) bands.
   Actin and myosin filaments show repeated organization pattern.
6. Intercalated disc (opposite I-band) unique. Dark staining lines crossing muscle fiber (zig zag) irregular intervals of cytoplasm. Two types of ICD—transverse and lateral.
7. Epimysium-dense, continuous fibrous skeleton of heart. Perimysium-enclose, muscle fascicule, endomysium-individual muscle fibers. Rich capillary network around muscle fibers.

III. SMOOTH MUSCLE (UNSTRIATED INVOLUNTARY PLAIN—VISCERAL)

1. Myocytes are small, length—15– 200 µm, diameter—3–8 µm, uterus—500 µm.
2. Fusiform or spindle in shape with broad central part and tapering ends.
3. The nucleus oval lies in central part of the cell.
   Cells are arrange so that thick central part of one cell is opposite to thin tapering end of adjoining cell.

4. Sacroplasm—dark eosinophilic, no cross striations and also no sacromere, but has fine longitudinal striations (obliquely placed actin—5 µm and myosin—2 µm. myofilaments).
5. Mitochondria, Golgi apparatus, ER and cytoskeleton.

Types of smooth muscles are two types

1. Unitary; a few nerves, and
2. Multiunitary; abundant nerves.

Clinical Correlation

1. Hypotrophy—enlargement of muscle fibers.
2. Skeleton muscle—exercise, cardiac muscle—left ventricular (hypertension), smooth muscle—uterus in pregnancy.
3. Regeneration—only in skeleton muscle.
4. Over action of smooth muscle—constriction of bronchi (asthma), colic (intestine, gall bladder, ureter)—relived by drugs.
5. Muscular dystrophy (dystrophin)—genetic disorder.
6. Proliferation of myofibroblast—in repair (cirrhosis of liver, fibrosis of lung or atheroma of arteries).

Nerve

NERVOUS SYSTEM

Nervous system controls and regulates both voluntary and involuntary activities of the body.

Function: Sensitivity, conductivity and responsiveness.

Nervous tissue is composed of neurons and neuroglial cells which are linked together in highly intricate manner and richly supplied by blood vessels: Neuropil cells of nervous system.

Two types of cells

a. Excitable cells—neurons are the functional unit

b. Non-excitable cells (neuroglia cells)—supporting and nutritive. Neuroglial cells are astrocyte, ependymal, oligodendrocytes and microglia.

Astrocyte: Star-shaped with number of processes radiating in all directions.

Two types of astrocyte

1. Protoplasmic astrocyte: Thick protoplasmic in the gray matter.

2. Fibrous astrocyte: Thin protoplasmic in the white matter (nutrition).

Oligodendrocyte (types 1–4) cells with a few processes. Myelination of axons in the brain and spinal cord (CNS) and enclose several axons. Proteins are different from that of Schwann cells.

Ependymal cells: Line the internal cavities or ventricles of the brain. Concerned with exchange between brain and CSF.

Microglia: Smallest cell with a few and short processes. Becomes active at the time of damage of the nerve tissue, i.e. phagocytosis.

Functions of Neuroglia

i. Provide mechanical support to neurons.

ii. Act as insulators between the neurons.

iii. Maintain suitable metabolic and ionic environment to the neurons.

iv. Repair of damaged nervous tissue.

v. Glial cells store neurotransmitters.

vi. Oligodendrocytes myelinate tracts (CNS). Schwann cells myelinate peripheral nerves.

vii. Ependymal cells exchange between brain and CSF.

Neurons are 120 μm in Diameter

These are excitable cells, i.e. reception integration, interpretation and transmission. Total number of neurons in the human brain is around 10^{12} (100 billions).

Neurons are two parts

a. Perikaryon (cell body) is a trophic center which transmits and receives stimuli.

b. Neurites:

  i. Dendrites (multiple and short afferent processes, which branch) and

  ii. Axon (single, long efferent process of uniform diameter).

Nucleus (5 μm)—single, central, vesicular with prominent nucleolus (owl's eye)

1. Binuclear in spinal and sympathetic ganglions.

2. Nucleus is envelop with two distinct layers with pores.

3. Chromatin fine, dispersed.

4. Sex chromatin (Barr body) is present in females.

Cytoplasm consists of Nissl bodies, mitochondrion, ribosome, Golgi apparatus, etc.

Nissl bodies—RER (stain intense with basic dyes). It is abundant and responsible for protein synthesis. Needed for:

1. Repair

2. Maintenance

3. Production of the enzymes

4. Neurotransmitters

Mitochondria—responsible for metabolic activity.

Golgi apparatus—large with secretory activity.

Neurofibrils (7–10 nm) are present in perikaryon and extend into the axon and dendrite stain: Cajal's method. Neurofibrils are distinctive feature of neuron, network permeating in cytoplasm. Concerned with transport of nutrition.

Dendrite—structurally resembles Perikaryon

1. Dendrites are unbranched or highly branched structures arise from cyton.

2. These carry impulse towards the cell body.

3. Dendrites are small and irregular, devoid of myelin sheath and are not insulated.

4. Nissl's granules are present and node of Ranvier absent.

5. Proteins MAP$_2$ present—immunochemical identification.

Axon—1 meter long and cylindrical

1. Axons starts from axon hillock and are branched at the tail ends.

2. They carry impulses away from the cyton.

3. These are long and uniform in size and may be myelinated or non-myelinated. Initial segment is non-myelinated.

4. Nissl's granules absent and node of Ranvier present.

Myelination of peripheral nerves (axons)

Axon invaginated in Schwann cell cytoplasm. Axon is suspended in the fold of cell membrane-mesoaxon. Mesoaxon becomes elongated spirals around the axon by several layers of cell membrane. Lipids are deposited between adjacent layers of the membrane. Layers of mesoaxon along with lipids form the myelin sheath, with thin outer most Schwann cell cytoplasm persists as neurilemma.

Peripheral Nerves

   i. Nerve fiber has an axon
  ii. Covered with axolemma (plasma membrane)
 iii. External, it is surrounded by myelin sheath with nodes of Ranvier.
  iv. Schwann cell cytoplasm sheath—neurilemma.
   v. Each nerve fiber—endoneurium (holds adjoining fibers) contains endothelial cells CF, RF fibroblasts and Schwann cells nucleus.
  vi. Number of nerve fibres form nerve fasciculus surrounded by perineurium, controls the diffusion of substance in and out of the axons.
 vii. Thin nerve has single nerve fasciculus.
viii. Number of fasciculi are held by dense connective tissue, epineurium that surrounds entire nerve. It contains fat that cushions the nerves. Loss of fat in bedridden patients lead to damage of the nerves which causes paralysis.

Schwann cell—supportive cells of peripheral nervous system (PNS)

- Myelination of nerve fibers of PNS.
- Myelin sheath provide insulation, protection and maintain the ionic environment of the axon.
- It is essential for vitality and phagocytic activity of axon.
- It influences the growth of the axons and responsible for regeneration and repair of the axon (PNS)
- Signals along the axons influence the proliferation and survival of the Schwann cells.

Applied Histology

1. Myelin sheath-around axon diameter. 1.5 μm (PNS) and 1 μm (CNS).
2. Large axons—thick myelination and greater internodal distance.
3. Myelination does not occur simultaneously in all axons.
4. Lipid metabolism disorders—myelination impaired.
5. Abnormal proteins form basis for neuropathies.

HISTOLOGY OF ANTERIOR HORN CELLS

Spinal cord: Transverse section. Stain: Silver impregnation (Cajal's method). Inner white and outer gray (H) matter.

Anterior Gray Horn (silver)

1. Motor neurons—multipolar and neuroglia.
2. Adjacent white matter, closed packed, myelinated axons.

Motor Neurons Multipolar

- Central vesicular nucleus and prominent nucleolus.
- Single non-myelinated axon and several dendrites.
- Cytoplasm—Nissl bodies.
- Nuclei of astrocyte and microglia.
- Blood capillaries
- Neuropil.

GANGLIONS

- Aggregations of cell bodies of the neurons outside the CNS (nucleus in CNS).

Ganglions are two types—sensory and motor

- Ganglions vary in size, small ganglion with few cell bodies and a large ganglion more than 50,000 cells.
- Each ganglion has connective tissue capsules

Cell bodies of neurons—dendrites and axons

- Neurons are surrounded by satellite cells

- Throughout the substances are fine collagen and reticular fibers.
- Blood capillary plexuses in between the meshes of nerve fibers.

1. Dorsal Root Ganglion or Spinal Ganglion on the Spinal Nerves; Located Outside the CNS; Pseudounipolar and Sensory Ganglion

1. Neurons are large, sensory, arranged in groups at peripheral (cortical) zone of ganglion.
2. Perikaryon 15–40 µm with central vesicular nucleus and prominent nucleolus. Cytoplasm rich in Nissl granules (basophilic) but not well defined and lipofusion pigments. Surrounded by two layers of capsular cells.
3. Cytoplasm—Nissl bodies and lipofusion pigments.
4. Numerous fascicles of nerve fibers pass between the neurons (non-myelinated and myelinated).

   Functional axons are slender pass into spinal cord and dendrites pass into the spinal nerve.
5. Rich blood capillaries within the mesh work of the nerve fibers.

2. Autonomic Ganglion: Sympathetic and Parasympathetic are Postganglionic

- Functional antagonists to each other. Supply smooth muscles of viscera, exocrine glands, blood vessels and sweat glands.

  Cell bodies are of multipolar motor neurons (H and E)
- Thick fibrous connective capsule envelops the ganglion.
- Neurons are stellate shape, smaller and multipolar.
- Neurons cell bodies are scattered in the ganglion.
- Perikaryon is 15–20 µm in diameter.
- Cytoplasm with well defined Nissl bodies, and in older individual's lipofusion pigments are present.

- Nucleus is eccentric vesicular with prominent nucleolus. Binucleated cells are common.

- Nerve cell bodies are not in groups in clumps but scattered through the ganglion among the non-myelinated and myelinated nerves.

- Capsular cells (satellite) around the neuron are not in uniform because neuron is multipolar. The nuclei in the stroma are of Schwann cells which are associated with neuronal processes that do not stain with H and E.

Circulatory System

The cardiovascular system provides a continuous circulatory system which is virtually closed. It permits blood vascular system to transport nutrients, oxygen, carbon dioxide, hormones, cells of immune defensive system to all parts of the body and remove the cellular products of metabolism. Responsible for gaseous exchange and temperature control of the body.

From the aorta, blood enters the arteries and arterioles. At the end, the arterioles are capillaries. The blood flows through the capillaries and enters the venous system.

The blood flows from the capillaries, to venules to veins to two largest veins, SVC and IVC.

Types of Circulation

    i. Systemic circulation.
   ii. Pulmonary circulation.
  iii. Portal circulation.
  iv. Lymphatic circulation (lymph from interstitial spaces between cells and veins.
   v. Circulations (others): CSF, perilymph and endocochlear fluids, ocular aqueous humor, synovial fluids and fluids of coelomic cavities.

THREE TUNICS OF BLOOD VESSELS

Tunica intima, tunica media and tunica adventitia.

Tunica Intima

Tunica intima has 3 layers from inside lumen to outside: Endothelium, subendothelium and internal elastic lamina.

Endothelium

Endothelium is the thin layer of flat cells that lines the inner surface of blood vessels forming an interface between circulating blood and the vessel wall. Cells of the endothelium are called endothelial cells or endotheliocytes.

It is only layer in the capillaries. Thereafter, addition of coats.Wide tile-like, curved to fit the curvature of blood vessel.

  i. Mononuclear, polygonal with sparse cytoplasm (squamous)
 ii. Endothelium serves major physiological roles.

Functions

- It provides smooth internal lining to the blood vessel and heart.
- It coated with glycocalyx which controls the transport across and contributes for non-thrombogenic properties of endothelium.
- It regulates the diffusion of substances.
- It secretes substances that provide vasodilatation and influences tone of smooth muscles.
- It produces clotting factors—controls coagulation.

Basic Structure of Arteries: Three concentric tunics

  i. Tunica intima (innermost)
 ii. Tunica media (middle)
iii. Tunica adventitia (outermost)

Tunica intima

  i. Endothelium, mononuclear, polygonal cells on the basal lamina.

ii. Subendothelium layer: Delicate fibroelastic connective tissue (CF, EF, smooth muscle and fibroblast cell)

iii. Internal elastic lamina: Band of elastic fibers.

Tunica media

- Chiefly consists of smooth muscle arranged circularly, between are elastic and collagen fibers. Limited by external elastic lamina.
- Thickest in arteries, thin in veins, absent in capillaries.

Tunica adventitia

i. Principally consists of connective tissue (CF, EF) run parallel to long axis of vessel.

ii. Prevents undue stretching or distension of the artery.

iii. It also contains vasa vasorum (supplies tunica adventitia and outer two-thirds of tunica media in case of arteries and all the tunicas in veins) and sympathetic nerves.

CLASSIFICATION OF ARTERIES

i. Large arteries (elastic arteries)—conducting vessels, e.g. aorta and its branches.

ii. Muscular arteries (medium sized arteries)—distributing vessels, with smooth muscles in tunica media.

iii. Arterioles—resistance arteries.

iv. Capillaries—exchange vessels.

1. Elastic arteries or conducting vessels (e.g. aorta, CCA, BrCT and SCA)

Tunica intima

i. 20% of total thickness. Endothelial cells flat, 1–2 μm thickness

ii. Subendothelial layer well developed (CF, EF, a few smooth muscle, fibroblast and macrophages—longitudinal orientation).

iii. Internal elastic lamina—1 μm. Thickness, difficult to identify.

Tunica media

It characterized numerous distinct elastic lamina or membrane 40–60 in number arranged concentrically and fenestrated. Also presents are CF, and smooth muscle + fibroblast cells. Each elastic lamina + adjacent intralaminar zone together is known as laminar unit.

Human aorta has 52 laminar unit. 11 um thickness. 60 EL → thoracic aorta, 30 EL—abdominal aorta. Number of elastic Lamina increases until 35 years.

At 50 years show degeneration replaced by collagen fibers. Limited by outer: external elastic lamina.

Tunica adventitia

It is thin not well developed. Consists of CF, EF and a few smooth muscles. Nutritive vessels vasovasorum, nerves bundles and lymphatic capillaries are present.

Tunica media of abdominal aorta prone for degenerative changes—aneurysm.

2. Medium sized arteries or muscular or distributing arteries

Most of arteries are muscular arteries. Wall is thick due to large amount of smooth muscles in tunica media. Distributing arteries because they distribute to different organs and regulate blood supply according to functional needs (contraction and relaxation of smooth muscles in tunica media), e.g. axillary, radial, femoral and popliteal arteries, etc.

Tunica intima—exhibits three definite layers

 i. Endothelial flat cells
 ii. Subendothelial layer delicates EF, CF, a few fibroblasts.
 iii. Internal elastic lamina very prominent, thick fenestrated band interwoven elastic fiber (folds—smooth muscles, tunica media seen only in postmortem).

Tunica media

Exclusively circular or helical dispersed smooth muscles cells (40 layers).

Between are small amount of connective tissue (CF, EF RF). External elastic lamina (marked).

Tunica adventitia

Often thick as tunica media. Dense irregular connective tissue (CF, EF) helically or longitudinal blending with neighboring tissue. Tiny vasa vasorum and nerves are present.

3. Arterioles—resistance vessels

Tunica intima

Only endothelium, no sub-endothelial layer. IEL—network of elastic fibers.

Tunica media

3–4 layers of thin circular smooth muscle, limited by EEL.

Tunica adventitia

Thick as tunica media contains CF, EF, arranged longitudinal, emerge surrounding tissues. Arterioles have relatively thick wall and narrow lumen. Control distribution of blood to capillary bed by vasoconstriction and vasodilatation. Their are prime controller of systemic blood pressure. Not involved in exchange. Regulated by sympathetic nerves.

4. Capillaries

Latin capillaries, from capillus means hair like, fine and slender. There are thin walled endothelial tubes, only one cell layer thick. Connect arteries with veins.

Terminal arterioles continue with capillary plexuses which vary tissue to tissue.

Capillaries are parts of microcirculation, these micro-vessels measuring (luminal diameter—8–12 um) slightly wider than RBCs.

Wall of capillaries

1. Single layer of endothelial cells, on basal lamina coated with glycoprotein.

2. Surrounded by thin delicate collagen fiber, reticular fiber.
3. Accompanied by pericytes, elongated undifferentiated cell.

Classification of capillaries

1. *Continuous capillary*
Continuous capillary (type I)—the individual endothelial cell lines the capillary lumen enough to encircle the entire lumen, e.g. muscles, lung, brain and skin.

2. *Fenestrated capillary*
Fenestrated capillary (type II)—the endothelial cell cytoplasm on each side of nucleus is perforated with pores or fenestrations closed by diaphragm, e.g. intestinal mucosa, endocrines and glomerular capillaries.

3. *Sinusoid (capillary)*
The capillaries endothelial cells exhibit some wide intercellular gaps which permit fluid exchange between plasma and the tissue fluid, e.g. liver, bone marrow, endocrine glands.

5. Medium sized vein femoral and axillary vein

Tunica intima
Endothelium, subendothelial and IEL are ill defined.

Tunica media
Thin compared to artery, small smooth muscle circularly. Tunica media well in lower limbs. Cerebral dural venous sinus—no smooth muscle.

Tunica adventitia
Well developed. Forms the bulk of the wall with longitudinal CF and a few smooth muscle. Vasa vasorum—supply all the three tunics and nerves.

6. Large vein (e.g. SVC, IVC and portal vein)

Tunica intima
Endothelial layer, subendothelial and IEL are ill defined.

Tunica media

Poorly developed with a few smooth muscles.

Tunica adventitia

Thickest and has 3 zones with vasa vasorum and nerves

    i. Dense fibroelastic connective tissue—spirally.

    ii. Middle-smooth muscle—longitudinal.

    iii. Outer zone—network of collagen fibers.

Applied Histology

Vasculitis is a feature inflammation of the blood vessels. Blood vessel inflammation is a painful condition that can have many possible causes.

Autoimmune disorders, tumors, leukemia, or certain medications have all been known to lead to inflamed veins and arteries.

Vasculitis, inflammation of veins (phlebitis) and arteries (arteritis).

Lymphoid System (Immune System)

Main function of lymphatic system or immune system to protect the individual from invading pathogens or antigens (bacteria, parasites or viruses).

Lymphatic system includes cells, tissues and organs that contain aggregation of immune cells, i.e. lymphocytes. It consists of:

- Lymphocytes T, B and NK cells
- Lymph vessels: Lymphatics
- Lymphatic organs
- Lymph-fluid

Development cells of lymphatic system—B, T lymphocytes and NK cells

Lymphocytes originate in embryo in the yolk sac → later reside in bone marrow (only site for stem cells) → divide and form lymphoblast → via blood circulation → thymus cortex and processed → T lymphocytes → enter blood stream and migrate to peripheral lymphatic tissues.

B lymphocytes undergo a phase of differentiation in bone marrow itself → migrates to peripheral tissues → plasma cells → secretes antibodies.

Primary lymphoid organs (central)

Thymus and bone marrow which have stem cells and lymphoblast bone marrow differentiates B lymphocytes. Thymus differentiates T lymphocytes.

Secondary lymphoid organs

Lymph node, spleen, tonsils, bone marrow, skin, MALT and GALT (Peyer's patches).

Common histological features of lymphatic organ

- Organ surrounded by connective tissue capsule (CF, EF, a few smooth muscle, fibroblast, macrophages, blood vessels and nerve fibers).
- Capsule sends—septa or trabeculae which divide parenchyma into cortex and medulla. Trabeculae carry blood vessels and nerves. Prenchyma made up of mesh work of reticular fibers and reticular cells (irregular star shape cells with many processes). Between cells and fibers are lymphatic sinuses (simple squamous epithelium, fenestrated).
- Lymphoblastic cell series and macrophages are entangled in the meshwork of RF and RC.
- Afferent and efferent lymph vessels are present.

Lymphatic cells arranged in three groups

1. Scattered free in the meshes of reticular framework.
2. Forms irregular cords of cells.
3. In form of rounded lymphatic nodules or follicles.

1. Lymph Node: Histology

Oval or bean shape, concavity-hilum through blood vessels (A and V) and efferent lymph vessels. Afferent lymph vessels enter through convex pericapsular adipose tissue.

1. Pericapsular adipose tissue: CF, EF and a few smooth muscle. Send trabeculae into node.
2. Two zones: Cortex (outer) and medulla (inner). Two zones no clear demarcation.
3. Several afferent lymph vessels enter capsule and efferent lymph vessels via hilum.
4. Cortex: Dark stain with dense packed lymphocytes. Several lymphatic follicles with germinal center.

5. Medulla: A few light lymphocytes. Framework RF and R cells with free lymphocytes (T and B).

Rich capillaries plexuses all over gland and dense around lymphatic follicle.

Lymph flow in node: Afferent lymph vessels→pierce the cortex → subscapsular sinus → cortical sinuses (trabeculae) → Medullary sinuses between medullary cords → efferent lymph vessels via hilum.

Function and applied

- Lymph node—produces, stores, recirculates and activates B and T lymphocytes.
- Filters lymph.
- Filtration of particles and microorganisms to keep them out of general circulation.
- Initiate immune response. Activation, proliferation of B and T lymphocytes.
- Infection—enlargement of lymph node. Inflammation—lymphadenitis.

2. Palatine Tonsil

Along the lateral wall of oropharynx, deep to mucous membrane. Traps bacteria and virus.

1. Consists of diffuse lymphoid tissue lymphatic follicles.
2. No afferent lymph vessel only efferent lymph vessels.
3. Covered by stratified squamous nonkeratinized epithelium on pharyngeal surface.

    Epithelium extends into the substance of invaginations and tonsillar crypts.
4. Other side of palatine tonsil is covered by hemicapsule (CF, EF). Capsule sends trabeculae into the tonsil.
5. Lymphatic follicles surrounded by lymph vessels→ efferent LV → pierce the hemicapsule and drain into deep cervical nodes.
6. Parenchyma has mucous glands open into crypts

7. Whole tonsil supported by delicate meshwork of collagen fibers and reticular fibers Connective tissue septa from capsule extend, forming partitions within the parenchyma. Follicles are on either side of septa.

8. No afferent lymph vessel, efferent lymph vessel → hemicapsule → superior constrictor → deep cervical lymph nodes.

Function and applied

- Select clones of B and T cells, revently invade the micro-organism.
- Antigens cross reticular epithelium results in immune function.
- Produces IgA and IgG—local and immediate protection of tonsil.
- B and T lymphocyte migrate from primary tissue and enters or leave the tonsil via blood stream.

Two classes of lymphocytes move to specific areas and proliferate when stimulated.

3. Spleen—Largest lymphoid organ present in abdominal cavity

It is encapsulated does not filter lymph but filters blood and phagocytose and destroys dead RBCs and other foreign bodies in blood. Spleen-naked eye-fresh shows red spots (red pulp) and white spots (white pulp). White pulp (immune function) and red pulp (filtration of blood, i.e. old RBCs).

1. Spleen covered by peritoneum, deep is thick capsule (CF, EF, a few smooth muscle and fibroblasts). Provides maturation of B and T lymphocytes in periarteriolar sheath.

2. Capsule sends trabeculae into substance. Main trabeculae enters through hilum and extends throughout organ. Trabeculae consists of trabecular arteries and veins. Spaces between trabeculae are reticular framework with RF, RC, B and T lymphocytes, macrophages, blood vessels and blood cells.

3. No cortex and medulla. No afferent and efferent lymphatic vessels.

4. Red pulp (75%)—venous sinusoids filled with blood, pulp arteries and venules. Between the sinusoids are splenic cords of Billroth (B and T lymphocytes, RF and RC and macrophage). Splenic tissue that consists of large venous sinuses → drain in splenic vein.

Venous sinuses separated by splenic cords of billroth (reticulum—RF, RE, T and B cells and macrophages).

Venous sinuses—50 μm diameter, lined by modified endothelial cells—Stave cells; fenestrated.

Splenic sinuses vascular spaces lined by a discontinuous layer of endothelial cells. Stave cells and supported by a fenestrated basal lamina. Surrounding cellular splenic cords provide a tissue framework.

5. White pulp (25%)—lymphoid follicles (B cells with germinal center) with small arteriole (eccentric), which dispersed whole of spleen lymphatic follicles with germinal C surrounding eccentric arteriole—malphigian corpuscle (0.25–1 mm, diameter). Small lymphatic cells proliferate when stimulated. Germinal center regress when infection subsides. Central A is a branch of trabecular A, unsheathed by lymphatic tissue.

6. Narrow marginal zone—between red and white pulp. Site of establishing immune response—splenic biology. Important in splenic biology—lymphocytes are free and plenty of antigens in venous sinus establish an appropriate immune responses.

7. Spleen has venous sinusoids, no lymph sinuses.

Splenic circulation: Close and open theory. Splenic A → trabecular A → central A (lose adventitia and ensheathed) by lymphoid follicle → penicillar A (red pulp) → ellipsoid A (surrounded reticular endothelial cells) → precapillary arteriole → venous sinusoids → venous system.

Functions

- Spleen filters blood and as RBCs, when passing through penicillar or ellipsoid A, aged cells get trapped and destroyed by macrophages.
- T and B lymphocytes multiple → immune competent.
- Enlarged spleen → splenomegaly increase lymphocytes—leukemia, destruction of RBCs: Malaria.

4. Thymus—Primary Lymphoid Tissue

Responsible for thymus processed T lymphocytes (80%)—immune system. Thymus present early childhood, atrophies at late adulthood. Provides unique microenvironment in which T cells precursors develop, divide and differentiate into clonal expansion and form mature T lymphocyte. Mature thymocytes leave thymus via bloodstream enter spleen, lymph node and other thymic dependent zones of lymphatic tissues.

Thymus has right and left lobes derived from III pharyngeal pouch (endoderm)

1. Each lobule surrounded by capsule which enters into interior and divide the thymus into incomplete lobules (medulla are continuous).
2. Each lobule—2 mm diameter.
3. Outer dark stain—cortex. Inner light zone-medulla which consists of two distinct cell lineage.

   T-cells and reticular cells (endoderm).
4. Cortex densely packed T lymphocytes, do not form lymphatic nodules.
5. Medulla, a few lymphocyte and more epitheloid RC and thymic corpuscles or Hassall corpuscles.

   Hassall corpuscles—balls of epithelial cells (30–100 µm) pinkish hyaline, exhibit central core-macrophages, cell debris and epithelial cells, surrounded by concentric layers of flattened epithelial cells—functional, not clear.

6. Lobules partially separated by connective trabeculae which contain blood vessels, nerves and efferent lymph vessels.

7. No afferent lymph vessel only efferent lymph vessels.

8. Thymocytes—stem cells in cortex derived from bone marrow. Epithelial cell (RE)—III PP (endoderm)—irregular eosinophilic, develop processes join similar protoplasmic of neighboring cells. Reticula (cellular) are maintain blood thymic barrier.

Function and Applied Histology

Myasthenia gravis: Tumor of thymus. Great weakness of skeleton muscles.

Treatment, removal.

Skin and its Appendages (Integumentary System)

Skin is the largest sensory organ of the body. It has an area of 2 square meters in adults, and weighs about 5 kg. Skin is the major barrier between the inside and outside of the body. It forms 16% of the total body weight. It covers the entire surface including EAM and the orifices of GIT, RS and UGT.

Human skin consists of two layers

1. Epidermis—ectoderm and avascular.
2. Dermis—mesoderm and highly vascular.

These two layers firmly adherent, varies in thickness (0.5–4 mm). Beneath dermis is hypodermis or superficial fascia.

Epidermis: Stratified squamous epithelium keratinized with distinct cell types in different layers. It is avascular. It consists of 5 layers.

Dermis: Dense irregular connective tissue with blood vessels, nerves, sweat and sebaceous glands. Thin skin has numerous hair follicles. It consists of two layers.

Junction between epidermis and dermis is markedly wavy. Finger like upward projections of dermis is dermal papilla. Downward projections of epidermis are epidermal papilla which interdigitate with dermal papilla.

Epidermis of Skin: Four types of cells

1. Keratinocytes is most dominant cell divide grow and migrate up and undergo cornification which forms protective surface of skin.

Other cells

2. Melanocyctes

3. Langerhans' cells

4. Merkel cells which are dispersed among keratinocytes in epidermis.

1. Thick skin has five distinct Layers: Epidermis

1. Stratum basale,

2. Stratum spinosum,

3. Stratum granulosum,

4. Stratum lucidum, and

5. Stratum corneum.

1. *Stratum basale* deepest with single layer of columnar or cuboidal cells (basement membrane). Stem cells undergo mitosis and give off keratinocytes to superficial layers. Produce keratin filaments—component of keratin.

2. *Stratum spinosum*—4–6 layers, keratinocytes. Shrink and appear as spines from surfaces (prickle cell layer). Synthesis of keratin filaments, assemble to bundles known as tonofilaments. They resistance to abrasion of epidermis.

3. *Stratum granulosum*—flat cells 1–5 layers deeply stained (basophilic) keratohyalin granules in cytoplasm. Granules contain filaggrin with tonofilaments together produce soft keratin of the skin. Nucleus condensed and pyknotic.

4. *Stratum lucidum*—it presents in thick skin. It is a homogenous, translucent, barely visible. Tightly packed flat cells, traces of nucleus and cell boundaries are not clear. Cells contain densely packed keratin filaments.

5. *Stratum corneum*—most superficial layer. Acellular, flat dead cells filled with soft keratin filaments (organelles and nucleus disappear). Squamous cells held together by lipid and carbohydrates, resistant to permeation to water.

Stratum basale and stratum spinosum are both germinative zone.

Stratum corenum, stratum lucidum, and stratum granulosum zone of keratinization or cornified zone. Stratum corenum is thick in palms and soles.

Dermis of skin (mesoderm) highly vascular, it binds epidermis

Dense irregular connective tissue contains epidermal derivatives: Sweat glands, sebaceous glands and hair follicles.

Dermis (thick)—Two Layers

1. Papillary layer—loose connective tissue fibers, capillary loops, fibroblasts, macrophages and tactile corpuscles.
2. Reticular layer—thick dense irregular connective tissue. No distinct boundary between two layers.

Two layers of dermis of thin skin, blends with hypodermis on which it rests withstand mechanical stress and provides support.

Dermis rich in blood vessels, nerves, lymph vessels, hair follicles, sweat and sebaceous glands.

Appendages of skin

1. Hair
2. Sebaceous glands with arrector pilorum muscle
3. Sweat glands with excretory ducts.

Thick skin—palms and soles: Sweat glands and ducts—no hair follicles

Epidermis: Stratum basale—single columnar cells with mitotic activity and melanocytes.

- Stratum spinosum (4–6 layers)—polyhedral cells with tonofilaments.
- Stratum granulosum—flat cells 1–3 layers keratohyalin granules in cytoplasm.
- Stratum lucidium—lightly stained flat cells with packed keratin filaments.
- Stratum corneum—wide layer of dead keratinized cells.

Dermis of thick skin—papillary and reticular layers.

- Dermal papillae are prominent in the papillary layer of the thick skin.
- Reticular layers dense irregular connective tissue, sensory meissner corpuscles, capillary loops, sweat glands with excretory ducts.

2. Thin skin covers most of the body. Epidermis is thin, presents hair follicles

Epidermis: Stratum basale—single columnar cells with mitotic activity: Stratum spinosum (4–6 layers)—polyhedral cells with tonofilaments. Stratum corneum—thin layer of dead keratinized cells.

Dermis of thin skin—papillary and reticular layers. It has the following:
1. Hair follicle
2. Sebaceous glands arrector pili muscles
3. Sweat gland (secretary) epidermis traversed by sweat gland duct
4. Arteriole and venules

Blood supply: From arterial plexus of superficial fascia. Secondary plexuses—dermis. Third plexuses—just below the dermal papilla. Capillary loops arise from this and pass to each papilla.

Epidermis derives nutrition entirely by diffusion. Rich sensory nerve supply: Dense network in dermis to various receptors.

Functions of the Skin

- Protection, sensory reception and excretion.
- Thermoregulation—sweat glands and arteriovenous anastomosis.
- Synthesis of vitamin D.
- Acts as physical barrier against entry of micro-organisms.
- Prevents loss of water from the body.
- Epidermis has pigments which protect from ultraviolet rays of sun.

Systemic Histology

Glands

Some epithelial cells in addition to secretion, excretion and absorption, manufacture specific substance known as glands.

1. Cells may be arranged in the form sheaths of epithelium with common secretary origin—mucous lining of stomach.
2. Cells arranged as highly folded configuration known as salivary glands.

Classification of glands

1. **Exocrine**—external secretary glands, secrete on surface via ducts.
   For example, GIT, RS, UGT their derivatives and skin.
2. Endocrine—ductless or internal secretary gland, secrete hormones directly into circulatory system that pass throughout the body for appropriate affects, e.g. thyroid, pituitary.
3. Paracrine glands are similar to endocrine, release products to perivascular plexuses which diffuse locally to target cells at immediate vincity.

Development of exocrine glands

1. Epithelial cell, multiply at site of future gland.
2. Cell mass grows into surrounding tissue as cords.
3. Deep part acquires lumen and outer zone forms secretary units.
4. Proximal part acquires lumen and becomes duct.

Developmen of endocrine gland: Deep secretary cells lose connection with surface and discharge hormones into the capillaries.

Exocrine glands are connected to exterior by ducts which discharge secretions, e.g.

- Salivary glands
- Liver
- Prostate
- Seminal vesicles
- Pancreas

End pieces or portio terminalis of terminal part of secretions.

Classification according to number of cells

i. Unicellular—single secretary cell. Interspersed among non-secretary epithelium, e.g. goblet
ii. Multicellular glands have many secretary cells in parenchyma discharge via large ducts, e.g. salivary glands.

According to number of ducts

i. Simple gland: Secretary cells discharge into one duct, e.g. sweat gland
ii. Compound gland: Groups of secretary cells. Each group discharges into own duct, which finally join to form excretory duct—open on surface, e.g. pancreas.

MULTICELLULAR GLANDS

These are simple and compound glands arranged in various ways.

i. Simple gland: All secretary cells discharge into one duct.

   Simple glands are acinar (alveolar) round, tubular, coiled tubular, branched tubular or alveolar type.
ii. Compound glands: Groups of secretary cells discharge into its own ducts. These ducts unite to form large excretory duct, ultimately drain into epithelial surface.

Compound glands: Acinar (alveolar), tubular alveolar and tubular type.

Classification according nature of secretions: Three types—(1) serous, (2) mucous and (3) mixed acini.

1. Serous Acini Secretions

1. Cells pyramidal on basement membrane
2. Lumen small
3. Cytoplasm—rich in granules eosinophil.
4. Nucleus oval and central.
5. Watery secretions
   For example, parotid and pancreas.

2. Mucous Acini—Secretions Contain Mucopolysaccharides

1. Cells are columnar.
2. Lumen visible.
3. Cytoplasm frothy (PAS) empty, mucinogen dissolved (H and E stains).
4. Nucleus is flat pushed to base.
5. Viscous and slimpy secretions.
   For example, globlet cells, sublingual gland.

3. Mixed Acini (Submandibular)—Mucous Acini with Serous Demilune

Classification according to modes of secretion poured

  i. Merocrine: Secretion by exocytosis (eccrine or epicrine) secretions of cell, extruded out without loss of other cellular products and cell remains intact, e.g. sweat gland.
 ii. Apocrine: Secretion by loss of cytoplasm. Microscopic apical portion is released along with secretion, e.g. mammary gland.
iii. Holocrine: Secretion through loss of entire cell or entire gland is disintegrated while discharging secretion, e.g. sebaceous gland.

Control of Secretions

- Most of exocrine glands vary in stages of synthesis, depletion except holocrine cells which die after release of their contents.
- Secretions are synthesized and stored until signaled to be released.
- Secretions are mainly under the parasympathetic or humoral.
  Cell rests before secretion.

Tumours of exocrine glands

- Benign—adenoma
- Malignant—adenocarcinoma

Major Salivary Glands: Parotid, Submandibular and Sublingual

Salivary glands discharge secretions into the oral cavity. Major salivary glands located some distance from the oral mucosa and connected by extraglandular ducts.

Minor glands lie in mucosa or submucosa open directly or by short ducts.

Salivary glands are modified epithelial structures which are separated from oral epithelium to manufacture, release and transport—salivary secretions.

All salivary glands are compound tuboalveolar (rasmose) secretary elements are known as end pieces or Portia terminalis.

- Parotid—purely serous.
- Submandibular mixed and predominately serous.
- Sublingual predominately mucous.

BASIC HISTOLOGY

1. All of these glands are compound tubuloacinar glands.
2. Salivary glands are covered by capsule which divides the gland into lobes and lobules.

3. Closed packed acini (serous or mucous or mixed acini)

4. Interlobular septa—ducts, blood vessels and nerves (parasympathetic and sympathetic)

5. Functionally the secretary acini can be divided into two groups:

   a. Serous acini with watery secretions, and

   b. Mucous secrete a very viscous product.

6. Ducts of the salivary glands—two parts.The ducts of the salivary glands according to their position in relation to the lobes and lobules.

   i. Interlobar ducts are embedded in the connective tissue surrounding the lobes, e.g. excretory ducts—stratified cuboidal epithelium with basal striations involved in electrolyte transport and intimate with blood capillaries.

   ii. Intralobular ducts are located inbetween the secretory acini within the lobules and surrounded by scanty connective tissue, e.g. intercalated ducts are cuboidal epithelium, striated ducts with columnar cells. Striations are found in the basal part of the cytoplasm of the cells.

7. Both secretory acini and intercalated duct are associated with myoepithelial cells, are basket shape interposed between basement membrane and cells. Contractions squeeze out secretions (ANS).

1. Parotid Salivary Gland: Features

1. Serous acini secretory units
2. Intercalated excretory duct
3. Striated excretory duct
4. Interlobular excretory duct
5. Interlobular connective tissue septa

2. Submandibular Salivary Gland (Mixed)

1. Serous acini
2. Mucous acini

3. Intercalated duct
4. Striated duct
5. Interlobular excretory duct
6. Interlobular connective tissue septa
7. Mucous acini with serous demilune.

3. Sublingual Salivary Gland (Mucus)

1. Lobules of the gland with mucous acini
2. Interlobular connective tissue septa
3. Interlobular excretory duct.

BLOOD SUPPLY AND NERVE SUPPLY

Salivary glands have rich blood supply. Arterioles and venules are present in interlobar connective tissue along with excretory duct. Capillaries present within the lobes and lobules around the acini.

Nerves: Parasympathetic nerves are secretory motor and sympathetic nerve are vasomotor.

Parotid: IX cranial nerve.

Submandibular and sublingual glands: VII cranial nerve.

FUNCTIONAL CORRELATION

Salivary gland produces 1 L/day of saliva enters the oral cavity via the main ducts.

Sailography—radio-opaque lipoid injected into the duct to identify ramification of duct system.

Histology of Respiratory System

Respiratory system consists of lungs and air passages. There are nasal cavities, pharynx, larynx, trachea, bronchi and bronchioles.

Conductive portion: That conducts air for gaseous exchange.

Extrapulmonary part is trachea and primary bronchi.

Intrapulmonary parts are secondary bronchi, tertiary bronchi (segmental), terminal bronchi, lobular bronchioles and terminal bronchioles.

Respiratory portion: That conducts air and also allows gaseous exchange. There are respiratory bronchioles, alveolar ducts → open into atrium → alveolar sacs → alveoli.

Functions

1. Main function exchange of gases and filtration of air, between lung and blood.
2. Regulation of pH.
3. Nonrespiratory functions secretion of immunoglobins, lysosomes and enzymes.
4. Secretes also vasoactive substances—angiotensin I which in pulmonary circulation → angiotensin II in lung.

1. Trachea: Wind Pipe—C6–T4 (10–12 cm)

D shape in CS (16–20 C shape hyaline cartilage). It is flexible membranous cartilaginous tube. Above trachea is continuous with larynx, below with primary bronchi and related posterior to oesophagus.

Histology of Trachea

It has four layers: (1) Mucous membrane, (2) submucosa, (3) hyaline cartilage with smooth muscle trachealis and (4) adventitia.

I. Mucous Membrane

1. Epithelium: Pseudostratified ciliated columnar (basal membrane).

   Epithelium has three types (LM) and 7 types (EM)

   i. Tall ciliated columnar cells (30%)—posses 200 cilia on each cell directed towards pharynx (12–16/min)

   ii. Goblet cells (28%)—secretes mucous traps dust particles which enter air passages → driven out by cilia. Able to divide and give rise to other cells. Present 6000–7000 mm^2.

   iii. Nonciliated columnar cells—secretes thin serous fluid, keeps surface epithelium moist and secrete IgA.

   iv. Brush cells—cuboidal cells with brush border (microvilli on luminal surface—sensory, chemo-receptor—afferent nerves).

   v. Kulchitsky cells (K cell) APUD, basal cells secretory granules infranuclear. Serotonin and histamine during hypoxia and regulates lobular growth, bronchial secretions and smooth muscle contraction.

   vi. Basal cells (30%)—stem cells, do not reach the lumen. Short cuboidal cells give rise to all types of cells.

   vii. Immature columnar cells—differentiate into ciliated columnar and goblet cells.

2. Lamina propria: Loose connective tissue with abundant arranged elastic fibers and diffuse lymphatic tissue associated with solitary lymphatic nodules.

3. Limited by longitudinal elastic membrane which separates lamina propria from submucosa.

II. Submucosa

It is below lamina propria. Loose connective tissue with plenty of elastic fibers, large blood vessels, lymphatic nodules and nerves (parasympathetic and sympathetic). Also tracheal glands: Serous and mucous.

Tracheal glands: Tubular serous, mucous and mixed-open into the lumen by ducts.

Serous keeps the epithelium moist. Mucous covers the epithelium and traps dust particles and moves towards the pharynx by the ciliary action.

III. Cartilage with Smooth Muscle Trachealis

i. Alters the shape and inserted into perichondrium.

ii. Hyaline cartilage is C shaped ends posterior and filled by trachealis muscle.

iii. 16–20 series of horse-shaped: Anterior two-thirds of rings.

iv. 1 mm thick and separated by interval of 4 mm.

v. First and last cartilage differs—thick and broad.

Hyaline cartilage consists of large chondrocytes (cell nests) at interior of cartilage, flatter at perichondrium. Enclosed by the perichondrium internal (convex) and external (flat). Cartilage calcified with age.

Function: It provides a semi-rigid supporting skeleton and prevent collapse of the airway passages, during inspiration.

Adventitia: Outermost fibroelastic connective tissue layer

i. External to the cartilage and its perichondrium and also trachealis.

ii. Dense connective tissue which blends with neighboring tissue and of consists of blood vessels, nerves (ANS), EF and mixed glands (serous and mucous) with plenty of adipose tissue.

2. Histology of Lung

Tubes become smaller and smaller

1. Epithelium: Height of epithelium reduced from tall ciliated columnar → cuboidal → simple squamous.
    i. Trachea, primary bronchi, secondary bronchi, terminal bronchi: Pseudostratified ciliated columnar.
    ii. Terminal bronchiole and respiratory bronchiole: Simple cuboidal.
    iii. Alveoli: Simple squamous epithelium.
2. Goblet cells: Diminish and disappear in bronchioles.
3. Glands: Present in bronchi and absent in bronchioles.
4. Cartilage rings in trachea and primary bronchi.
5. Cartilage plates: Secondary, tertiary bronchi, absent in bronchioles.
6. Smooth muscle:
    i. Posterior in trachea
    ii. Secondary, tertiary bronchi: Encircles between mucous membrane and submucosa.
    iii. Bronchioles between mucous membrane
7. Adventitia: Elastic fibers are present.

Lung (panoramic view): Stain

Intrapulmonary bronchi (secondary, tertiary): Bronchioles (lobular, terminal, respiratory), alveolar ducts and alveoli.

1. Intrapulmonary bronchi

These are five layers
 i. Mucous membrane, smooth muscle, submucosa, cartilage plates and adventitia.
    Intrapulmonary bronchus: Mucous membrane— pseudostratified ciliated columnar + 7 types of cells.
 ii. Smooth muscle encircles entire lumen between mucous membrane.
 iii. Submucosa with bronchial glands.

iv. Cartilage plates—several, surround between submucosa and adventitia

v. Adventitia—connective tissue, bronchial vessels, lymphatic nodules and nerves.

2. Intrapulmonary bronchi (secondary and tertiary)

i. Mucous membrane: Seven types (epithelium pseudostratified ciliated columnar + lamina propria).

ii. Smooth muscle encircles between MM and SM.

iii. Submucosa—bronchial glands (serous and mucous).

iv. Cartilage plates—encircles between SM and adventitia.

v. Adventitia—connective tissue blood vessels, nerves and lymphatic nodules.

3. Terminal bronchiole

i. Mucous membrane (four types of cells)
   a. Simple ciliated cuboidal or columnar cells
   b. Clara cell (bronchiolar cells) secretes, surfactant decreases surface tension, also a stem cell
   c. Brush cell (chemoreceptor)
   d. K cell (serotonin) no goblet cells

ii. Smooth muscle surrounds the lamina propria. Lumen shows mucosal folds (contraction).

iii. Adventitia: It consists of blood vessels, nerves, bronchiolar macrophages + are phagocytic because cilia are absent.

Terminal bronchioles

i. Mucous membrane: Four types (epithelium—simple cuboidal, clara cells, B and K) + lamina propria.

ii. Smooth muscle encircles between MM and adventitia.

iii. Adventitia—connective tissue, blood vessels, nerves and lymphatic nodules.
   Submucosa and cartilage plates are absent

4. Respiratory bronchiole

Gaseous exchange occurs. Respiratory bronchiole → lung unit. Are short branching tubes 4 mm long and 0.5 mm diameter. Branch into several alveolar duct.

1. Simple cuboidal epithelium with Clara cells surrounded by
2. Smooth muscles, elastic fibres (EF) and blood vessels and nerves.

5. Alveolar ducts

Cone shape, 2 million in each lung

i. Simple squamous epithelium,

ii. Fibroelastic connective tissue

Alveolar ducts terminate in atria (polygonal or hexagonal) from which arise alveoli sacs (multilocular) and alveoli—parenchyma of lung.

6. Alveoli

Alveoli form the parenchyma of the lung. Polygonal or hexagonal, tightly packed that does not have separate wall. IAS-delicate wall with extensive capillary network and elastic follicle. Alveolar walls: Interalveolar septa (IAS).

Alveoli epithelium is spongy alveolar capillary barrier (air blood barrier) 1.5 µm.

It consists of: Type I pneumocyte, type II pneumocyte, alveolar macrophages (dust cells), IAS: Endothelial cell of capillaries and Brush cells.

Applied Histology

During the pulmonary congestion the dilated capillaries, leakage of blood into the alveolar spaces. Brown granules of hemosiderin from breakdown of RBCs appear in the macrophage cytoplasm. These macrophages are sometimes called 'heart failure cells' because of their association with congestive heart failure.

Histology of
Gastrointestinal Tract (GIT)

TONGUE HISTOLOGY

Fibromuscular organ present in oral cavity and oropharynx. Dorsal and ventral surfaces, attached to floor. Body, root, apex (tip) and 2 lateral margins. Dorsal surface → posterior 1/3rd and anterior 2/3rds by sulcus terminalis, apex → foramen caecum.

Tongue

It consists:
1. Core of striated muscle fibers runs in all directions and interlacing, supported by connective tissue.
   - Muscles run in vertical, transverse and longitudinal direction.
   - Intricate movements of tongue → chewing and swallowing of food.
2. Perimysium of muscle consists of fibroelastic, large vessels, nerves (sensory and motor) and adipose tissue.
3. Tongue covered by mucous membrane—stratified squamous non-keratinized epithelium.

Ventral Surface

1. Smooth mucous membrane: Stratified squamous non-keratinized epithelium also lines the rest of oral cavity.
2. Deep is lamina propria consists of fibroelastic tissue, blood vessels, lymph vessels, nerves and salivary glands.
3. Skeletal muscles (intrinsic)
   Submucosa is absent.

Dorsal Surface

1. Mucous membrane irregular and rough due to elevations.
2. Anterior 2/3rds show numerous projections, called papillae. Filiform, fungiform, foliate (absent) and circumvallate.
2. Posterior 1/3rd shows numerous elevations due to lymphoid tissue deep to epithelium, i.e. lingual tonsils.

Histology of dorsal surface

1. Dorsal surface (irregular) associated with papillae and lined by stratified squamous non-keratinized epithelium.
2. Deep to the epithelium is lamina propria consisting of the fibroelastic tissue with blood vessels, lymph vessels, nerves and anterior salivary glands.
3. Skeletal muscles (intrinsic).

Submucosa is absent

Anterior 2/3rds or oral part of the dorsum of the tongue.

Four types of papillae with taste buds

  i. Filiform is smallest and no taste buds. The filiform papilla is one of four types of lingual papillae, and its function is purely mechanical; it has no sensory structures.
 ii. Fungiform
iii. Foliate—absent in humans, which are most easily seen in the rabbits and hares.
 iv. Circumvallate is largest in front of sulcus terminalis.

 Remaining types of lingual papillae are sensory in function (taste buds). They include:

 Posterior 1/3rd pharyngeal part of the dorsum of tongue:
1. Epithelium is stratified squamous non-keratinized, sends crypts into underlying lymphatic tissue.
2. Lamina propria contains lymphatic follicles (lingual tonsil) some with germinal center.

3. Crypts remain clean unlike palatine tonsil because underlying mucous glands (posterior lingual glands) open into bottom of crypts.
4. Skeletal muscles—intrinsic.

Lingual Glands in the Lamina Propria

These are serous, mucous and mixed, numerous in post-sulcal region, a few in margins and apex.

  i. Mucous glands → pharyngeal part (posterior lingual glands).
 ii. Serous glands (von Ebner) in relation circumvallate papilla open in vicinity of taste buds.
iii. Serous and mucous (mixed) glands → largest on ventral aspect of apex (anterior lingual glands).

Function: Dissolve the substance to be tasted, spread it over the taste buds and wash away after it is tasted.

Taste buds present on circumvallate and fungiform papillae, soft palate, epiglottis, and palatoglossal arch.

Tongue: Taste buds → nerve supply

Anterior 2/3rds → VII, posterior 1/3rd → IX and root → X. All nerves lose myelin before they reach taste bud.

Tongue: Points to Remember

- Ventral surface → smooth mucous membrane.
- Dorsal surface → mucous membrane irregular.
- Anterior 2/3rds shows numerous projections called papillae (filiform, fungiform and circumvallate with taste buds).
- Posterior 1/3rd shows numerous elevations→lingual tonsils
- Mucous membrane stratified squamous nonkeratinized epithelium.
- Deep to epithelium is lamina propria consists of fibro-elastic tissue consists of blood vessels, lymph vessels, nerves and salivary glands.
Skeletal muscles, intrinsic.

GENERAL FEATURES OF GIT

Starts from oral aperture and ends at anal aperture. Mature gut wall presents laminated structure with four main layers which are firmly attached to each other, boundaries are clear. There are variations in the lining epithelium, it includes four "tunics" which have subdivisions:

1. Mucous membrane has 3 strata

a. Lining epithelium

b. Lamina propria

c. Muscularis mucosa (smooth muscle)

2. Submucosa: Strong and highly vascular connective tissue and nerve plexuses.

3. Muscularis externa: Inner circular and outer longitudinal smooth muscles.

4. Serosa/adventitia.

1. Oesophagus: Histology

C_6-T_{10}, 25 cm (10") muscular tube, extends pharynx to stomach, behind trachea.

Mucosa of oesophagus is exposed to various mechanical injuries due to rough materials swallowed. It is lined by multilayered epithelium (protects). It is lined by non-keratinized stratified squamous epithelium in humans. Epithelial cells renewed 2–3 weeks.

Esophagus showing four layers: Food passes rapidly through esophagus—(1) mucosa, (2) submucosa, (3) muscularis externa and (4) adventitia.

I. **Mucous membrane:** Thick, pinkish above, pale yellow below (live).

Mucous membrane presents several longitudinal folds, disappear when distended.

Epithelium: Protective, non-keratized stratified squamous epithelium. Thick—300–500 μm.

1. Epithelium is stratified squamous non-keratinized epithelium. Keratohyalin granules may be present in some of the surface cells.

   Basal cells—columnar, middle-cuboidal, superficial-flat cells → migrate from deep to superficial → 1 week

   Occasional melanocytes, entero-endocrine (APUD), and Langerhans cells, present.

2. Lamina propria: Thin connective tissue, no glands except in abdominal part (cardiac glands).

   Finger-like pegs are acellular projections papilla project into the epithelium.

   Prevent separation of epithelium from the underlying connective tissue.

3. Muscularis mucosa is quite prominent.

   i. It is absent in upper part

   ii. Middle part, it is mainly longitudinal progressively thicker

   iii. Lower part, it is plexiform.

II. **Submucosa:** Moderately dense irregular connective tissue.

Special features:

1. Tubuloalveolar mucous secreting glands are scattered throughout the submucosa of the esophagus. Most frequent at the level of bifurcation of trachea. Ducts pass through MM and LP and open into oesophagus lumen.

2. Small lymphatic aggregation at lower part. Large blood vessels and submucosal nerve plexuses (Meissner).

III. **Muscularis externa:** Inner circular and outer longitudinal.

1. Upper third of the esophagus contains skeletal muscle.

2. Middle third has both skeletal and smooth muscle.

3. Lower third—entirely of smooth muscle.

The muscle bundles in each layer are separated by connective tissue and are well vascularized by blood vessels and myenteric nerve plexus.

IV. **Adventitia:** Of the esophagus surrounds the muscularis externa.

Serosa: In the abdominal part.

2. Stomach: Histology

There are three regions: Cardiac, fundus and body (identical histology), pylorus. Mucous membrane (special) epithelium, penetrates into LP as gastric pits, submucosa, muscularis externa (special) and serosa.

I. Mucous Membrane

1. **Lining epithelium:** Simple columnar epithelium secretes mucous (lubricant protect, against acids and enzymes produced by mucous itself). Mucous cells also produce blood group factors.
2. **Lamina propria:** Studded with long tubular gastric glands which open on the base of the pits.
    i. Gastric pits (tubular infoldings of surface epithelium 1/4th in F and B, 2/3rds in pylorus) are lined by simple columnar epithelium and extend into the lamina propria.
    ii. Gastric glands—simple tubular located below the epithelium descend into lamina propria up to MM and 3–7 glands open at base of pit.

Three types of gastric glands

a. Principal glands (F and B)
b. Cardiac glands
c. Pyloric glands

Main or principal gastric gland: Five types of cells

1. Chief, zymogen or peptic cells: Digestive enzymes.
2. Oxyntic or parietal cells (gastric acid and HCl) give beaded appearance.

3. Mucous neck cells: Chemical different from mucous secreted by lining cells (neutral mucous). These cells produce acid mucous.
4. Enteroendocrine cells (GP system or argentaffin cells, take up silver stains): These are pyramidal cells with clear cytoplasm. Secrete gastrin, serotonin and somatostatin have paracrine effect (capillaries).
5. Undifferentiated cells—neck or isthmus and precursor cells.

Gastric gland (simple or branched) is divided into base, neck (middle) and isthmus.

- Isthmus—parietal and chief cells
- Neck—mucous, parietal and stem cells
- Basal—chief, parietal, and EE cells

Lamina propria: Like in all regions with connective frame work—CF, EF, RF, reticular cells.
3. Muscularis mucosa: Layers → well developed, inner circular and outer longitudinal, additional circular outer-most. Inner circular end strands between glands—contraction helps emptying.

II. Submucosa

Connective tissue, large blood vessels, lymph vessels, and ganglionic nerve plexus (Messiener and Henle).

III. Muscularis Externa

Well developed and oriented into 3 layers, inner—oblique, middle—circular and outer—longitudinal. Auerbach/ myenteric plexus between inner circular layer and innermost oblique layer. Causes between churning and mixes food with gastric secretions.

IV. Serosa

Thin layer of connective tissue overlies muscularis externa covered by simple squamous epithelium. Blood vessels, nerves, lymphatic and adipose tissue.

3. Small Intestine: Histology

Extends from the pyloric orifice of the stomach to the ileocaecal orifice. It is 120 cm or 5 meters in length, coiled in the abdomen. Duodenum—25 cm, jejunum (2 meters)—2/5th and ileum (3 meters)—3/5th.

General pattern: Mucosa, submucosa, muscularis externa and serosa.

1. **Specialization of mucosal surface:** Thick and vascular—proximal part, thin and less vascular—distal part.
2. Plica circularis, villi and microvilli which increase the area for absorption of nutrients and fluids.
3. Villi (0.5–1.5 mm long). Evagination of epithelium.
4. Crypts of Liberkühn (0.3–0.5 mm) are packed, deep tubular invaginations of epithelium into lamina propria and are intestinal glands open into bases of villi. Epithelium of crypts continuous with the villi. Crypts are invaginations of epithelium into the lamina propria. It is lined with the epithelium which is continuous with villi.
5. **Microvilli:** Tall columnar absorptive cells are covering the villi, have striated border
   1. Increase surface area for absorption in 20 folds.
   2. Assist digestion of enzymes.

I. Epithelium

1. Lining epithelium covers the villus

Epithelium is striated border (microvilli): Four types of cells

1. Enterocytes: Tall columnar cells with striated border.
2. Goblet cells.
3. Enteroendocrine cells.
4. Microfold (M) cells migrating lymphocytes.

Epithelium covering the crypts or intestinal glands: Five types of cells:

1. Paneth cells
2. Stem cells—bases of crypt
3. Enteroendocrine cells
4. Goblet cells
5. Caveolated cells (chemoreceptor)

2. **Lamina propria:** Connective tissue provides mechanical support for epithelium. Extends between intestinal glands and into core of villi. RF, rich blood capillaries, nerve fibers and smooth muscle.

   Ileum: Aggregations of lymphatic tissue (Peyer's patches).

3. **Muscularis mucosa:** Inner circular and outer longitudinal. Follows surface profiles of circular folds and sends slips into core of villi.

II. Submucosa: Connective tissue, blood vessels, lymphatics and Meissner's plexus form core in plica circularis.

   Duodenum: Brunner glands (mucosal), open bases of crypt (largest at pyloric end and diminish at DJ junction). Brunner glands: Mucous glands—alkaline (rich in bicarbonate) neutralize acid secretions of stomach.

III. Muscularis externa: Thin, outer longitudinal and inner thick, circular.

IV. Serosa: Peritoneum containing subserous stratum loose connective tissue.

Duodenum: Adventitia (posterior).

Duodenum

1. *Mucosa*

   Villi—broad tongue-like with intestinal glands in lamina propria.

   Villi—enterocytes with microvilli and goblet cell.

   Crypts of Lieberkühn—Paneth, stem cells and EE.

2. *Submucosal*—Brunner's glands.

3. *Muscularis externa*—inner circular and outer longitudinal layers of smooth muscle

4. *Serosa/adventitia*

Jejunum

1. *Mucosa*

Villi—leaf-like with intestinal glands in lamina propria. Villi—enterocytes with microvilli and goblet cell. Crypts of Lieberkühn—Paneth stem cells and EE.

2. *Submucosa*—connective tissue.

3. *Muscularis externa*—inner circular and outer longitudinal layers of smooth muscle.

4. *Serosa*.

Ileum

1. *Mucosa*

Villi—finger-like with intestinal glands in lamina propria. Villi—enterocytes with microvilli and goblet cell. Crypts of Lieberkühn: Paneth stem cells and EE.

Lamina propria—Peyer's patches (M cells) extend submucosa and muscularis mucosa.

2. *Submucosa*—connective tissue.

3. *Muscularis externa*—inner circular and outer longitudinal of smooth muscle.

4. *Serosa*.

4. Large Intestine: Histology

It measures—140–150 cm. Starts caecum and vermiform appendix → ascending colon → transverse colon → descending colon → rectum and anal canal.

Function: Absorption of water and electrolytes and formation of faeces.

Plica circulares absent, only temporary folds, absence of villi, absence of Paneth cells.

Presence of plenty of goblet cells and tall columnar cells with striated border. Lamina propria is thick, with solitary lymphoid follicles.

I. **Mucous membrane:** Pale, smooth and colon show numerous cresentic folds.
Epithelium (no villi), intestinal glands (crypts), lamina propria with lymphatic nodules and mucous membrane.

1. Surface epithelium: Five types of cells

1. Tall columnar cells with microvilli (striated) vacuolated absorptive cells. Secrete mucus and antibodies (IgA → provide protection).
2. Goblet cells abundant secrete mucus that is lubricant and facilitates the passage semisolid contents of colon. Number increases as proceeds caudally.
3. Microfold (M) cells—triangular cells with microfolds lying over lymphatic follicle.
4. Enteroendocrine cells
5. Brush cells—columnar cells with apical tuft of microvilli and sensory cells.

2. Intestinal glands

1. Short columnar cells (EE)—absorptive cells.
2. Goblet cells inbetween EE cells.
3. Stem cells at bases of crypts with pericyclic mitotic changes.

3. Lamina propria (supportive) connective tissue surrounds the glands and specialized fibrous tissue around solitary lymphoid follicles (abundant in caecum, appendix and rectum).
4. Muscularis mucosae—prominent, inner circular and outer longitudinal.

II. **Submucosa:** Dense irregular connective tissue with numerous blood vessels, Meissner nerve plexus and lymph vessels. Contain fat cells (PAS)—muciphages (more in rectum).

III. **Muscularis externa:** Colon is modified smooth muscle. Inner circular muscle layer is continuous in colon wall, whereas the outer muscle is condensed into three broad longitudinal bands, called *Taeniae coli*.

IV. **Serosa:** Transverse and sigmoid colon and attached to the body wall by a mesentery which contains loose CT, adipocytes, blood vessles and nerve plexus. Ascending and descending colon are retroperitoneal and their posterior surface is the adventitia.

5. Vermiform Appendix

Narrowest part of colon, inflammation is known as appendicitis.

Histology similar to colon (large intestine): Mucosa, submucosa, muscularis externa and serosa. Lumen is narrow thrown three folds or horns.

Mucous membrane: Epithelium-like colon (simple columnar cell) with goblet cells.

Lamina propria—crypts poor developed.

Mucous membrane—broken (lymphoid tissue).

Submucosa contains abundant lymphoid tissue which fills it.

Muscularis externa: Inner circular and outer longitudinal which are complete with myenteric plexus.

Serosa: Complete coat consists of blood vessles, nerves and adipose cells.

LIVER: HISTOLOGY

Liver (reddish brown largest gland) in the body 1.5 kg and is located in the right upper quadrant of the abdomen.

Liver consists of complex network of epithelial cells, hepatocytes.

Hepatocytes, the epithelial cells perform both endocrine and exocrine

1. Formation and secretion of bile.
2. Storage of glycogen, fat and vitamins.
3. Synthesis of urea.
4. Synthesis and secretion of many plasma proteins, including clotting factors.

5. Metabolism of cholesterol and fat.

6. Detoxification of many drugs and other poisons.

7. Processing of several steroid hormones.

8. Catabolism of hemoglobin from worn-out red blood cells.

Histology

1. Glisson capsule send extensions into liver substance dividing into lobules: Hepatic lobules roughly hexagonal in shape.

2. Connective septa carry branch of hepatic A, tributary of portal vein and bile ductule → portal tract or canal consists portal triad.

3. Parenchyma of hepatic lobules (hexagon). It composed of cells arranged in anatomizing plates or cords—hepatic lamina. Between plates are vascular spaces—hepatic sinusoids.

4. Portal triad (PV, HA and BD) at the angles. Blood from the portal vein and hepatic A enters the sinusoids between the hepatic cords of cells → central vein. Bile → collected by bile canaculi between cell membrane of hepatocytes. Flow of bile opposite to the flow of blood.

5. Hepatocytes are highly versatile action. Its major metabolic activities are assisted by Kupffer cells (hepatic macrophages) line the sinusoids phagocytic, storage and supportive.

Classical hepatic lobulation of liver structural and functional unit

  i. Each lobule is typically hexagonal and is centered central vein. Lobules are distinctly demarcated by connective tissue. In human liver lobules emerge with one another.

  ii. Within each lobule, hepatocytes are arranged in form of hepatic cords separated by adjacent sinusoids.

  iii. Hepatic cord and lamina one cell thickness branch and form network. Hepatic cord extends from central vein to peripheral. Between are sinusoids. Each lobule an angular intervals with connective tissue.

iv. Portal canals contain:

1. Tributary of portal vein
2. Branch of hepatic A
3. Interlobular bile duct
4. Lymph vessel (not visible)
5. Nerve plexus.

v. Portal triad: Tributary of portal vein (largest tubule), branch of hepatic A (II large tubule, 3 tunics) and interlobular bile duct (smallest—cuboidal epithelium) lymph vessel (not visible) and nerve plexus (ANS).

vi. Sinusoids are lined fenestrated endothelium. Lies adjacent to hepatic cords with no intervening connective tissue, so that each hepatocyte is bathed by blood plasma interposed amongst endothelial cells are hepatic macrophages—Kupffer cells.

vii. Portal lobule—nutritional unit of liver: Area of liver tissue comprising parts of three adjoining hepatic lobules. It may be triangular or hexagonal, supplied by one tributary of portal vein. Portal traid is central point and with three central veins at tips of angle.

viii. Portal acinus of Rapaport: It is a metabolic unit of liver (small unit). It is diamond-shape of liver parenchyma supplied by one hepatic arteriole. Two central veins lie at the end of acinus and hepatic A as central axis.

Clinical Correlation

- Liver performs hundreds of function.
- Hepatocyte performs more functions than any other cells in the body and they play both endocrine and exocrine roles.
- Exocrine—bile.
- Endocrine—role in carbohydrate, protein and fat metabolism.
- Storehouse—glucose, lipids, vitamins, etc.
- Detoxifies—drugs and alcohol.

PANCREAS: HISTOLOGY

It is soft, lobulated grayish pink across the posterior abdominal wall.

It has exocrine part of the enzymes into pancreatic duct → II duodenum.

Endocrine parts, the hormones into blood capillaries.

Exocrine part: Main mass compound tuboacinar serous cells—secrete pancreatic juice, regulated by intestinal hormones (EE) and vagus nerve (parasympathetic).

Endocrine part: Islets of Langerhans scattered among secretory acini. Acini are arranged as pale stained units. One million islets—tail of pancreas.

1. Pancreas is surrounded by delicate capsule. Septa extend from the capsule into gland → divide into number of lobes and lobules separated by interlobar septa.
2. Lobules are packed serous acini and ducts, group of islets separated by plenty of delicate connective tissue consists of blood vessels, lymph vessels, nerves (ANS) small ganglion.
3. Packed secretory acini cells with scattered islets cells within the lobules. Islets are surrounded rich capillary net work. Secretory serous acini are long, tubular or pear shape closely packed. Islets are pale staining.
4. Serous acini: Composed 5–8 pyramidal cells around small lumen with centroacinar cells in the center belong to duct system, i.e. intercalated duct cells invaginated into secretory units. Serous acinar cells with triangular with round nucleus. Cytoplasm: Basophilic, acidophilic zymogen granules. Between acini are delicate connective tissue. Myoepithelial cells are absent.
5. Duct system: Secretions are poured
   1. Centroacinar
   2. Intercalated duct (cuboidal)
   3. Intralobular duct (cuboidal)
   4. Interlobar ducts (tall columnar with striated border)
   5. Main pancreatic duct (stratified cuboidal cells).

6. Lobes separated by interlobar connective tissue blood vessle, nerves (ANS) and ganglions, lymphatics and large interlobar duct (stratified cuboidal).
7. Islets of Langerhans: Spheroidal or ellipsoid clusters. Each islets is separated from acinar cells by thin reticular tissue and it is surrounded by dense blood capillaries.

   Six types of cells: Alpha or a cells, beta cells, delta or D cells, D1 cells, C cells and PP(F) cells.

Gallbladder

On the inferior surface of liver, hollow muscular organ, stores and concentrates bile, absorbs H_2O and adds mucoid substance. It receives and stores bile from the liver via the hepatic and then cystic duct. It presents three layers:

1. Mucosa (highly folded-temporary)—mucous membrane variable branching folds, look like villi, except that vary in size, shape and irregular arranged.
   i. Epithelium—tall columnar with brush border, no goblet cells. Neck region has tubuloalveolar mucus glands that secrete neutral mucin and contain neuroendocrine cells.
   ii. Lamina propria—thin loose areolar tissue.
2. Fibrous muscularis layer: Bundles of smooth muscle fibers arranged in circular, oblique and longitudinal direction with elastic and collagen fibers interlacing with muscles. Surrounded by perimuscular connective tissue.
3. Serosa/adventitia on free surface. Perimuscular connective tissue composed of collagen, elastic tissue, fat, vessels, lymphatics, nerves.

   No muscularis mucosa or submucosa.

Urinary System

HISTOLOGY OF KIDNEY

Kidney as vital function

1. Maintains homeostasis.
2. Regulate blood pressure, blood electrolytes and blood volume.
3. Maintains acid–base balance.
4. Produces two hormones—renin and erythropoietin.
   - Ureters convey the urine from the kidney to urinary bladder.
   - Urinary bladder stores the urine until it is voided.
   - Urethra transports the urine to exterior.

Kidneys are Bean-shaped in Lumbar Region

Two surfaces: Anterior and posterior, two borders: Lateral and medial.

Two poles: Upper and lower.

Medial border presents hilum through which passes blood vessels (A and V) and ureter.

Hilum leads to renal sinus (fat filled space) which is occupied by upper end of ureter—renal pelvis.

Renal pelvis divides 2 or 3 major calyces.

Each major calyx divides number of minor calyces (7–12 in each kidney).

MACROSCOPIC STRUCTURE OF KIDNEY (CORONAL SECTION)

Outer cortex is granular and dark due to RC, RT (PCT and DCT).

Inner medulla is striated and light due to loop of Henle, CD and PD.

Functional unit of kidney (uniferous tubules): Two parts:

1. Nephron: Secretory part develops from metanephros.
2. Collecting part develops from ureteric bud.
   1–4 millions of nephrons present in each kidney.

Nephron (secretory part)

It consists of:

1. Renal corpuscle—glomerulus and Bowman's capsule (filtration of plasma)
2. Renal tubules—PCT, loop of Henle and DCT (selective reabsorption and filtration).

Collecting part consists of: 1. Collecting duct and 2. papillary duct.

Renal medulla

It consists of:

1. Renal pyramids (8–18) striated, pale and triangular conical masses
2. Renal columns—tissue between the renal pyramids.

Renal cortex is granular

It consists of mainly nephrons. Each kidney has 1–4 million functional units of nephrons.

Lobe of kidney: Each pyramid associated with overlying cortex.

1. Microscopic of Kidney

Cortex

1. Renal corpuscles (glomerulus and Bowman's capsule).
   Renal corpuscle (150–250 µm) rounded epithelial lined

with tuft of capillaries. Present in cortical arches and a few in renal columns.

Filtration of plasma: It Consists of

a. Glomerulus: Tuft of capillaries. Characteristic of cortex: Rounded tuft of anatomizing blood capillaries united at both ends to afferent and efferent arterioles: Vascular pole of nephron. AA—branch of interlobular artery → capillaries plexuses → EA (not vein). AA is double size of EA, lumen is equal (hydrostatic pressure).

b. Bowman capsule—double layered with narrow space covering capillaries. Bowman capsule encloses the capillaries.

   1. Double layer separated by urinary space.
   2. Outer parietal layer: Simple squamous epithelium.
   3. Inner visceral layer: Podocytes (stellate cell with process).
   4. Urinary space continuous with lumen of renal tubule, i.e. PCT at urinary pole.

2. **Convoluted tubule: PCT, DCT**

   i. PCT (60 µm) tortuous is most numerous in cortex. Small lumen lined simple cuboidal epithelium, eosinophilic granules in cytoplasm and brush border (microvilli)—selective reabsorption of filtrate. Initial part is convoluted present in cortex.

   Terminal part—straight—descends in medulla.

   ii. DCT (30 µm)—a few in cortex. Large lumen cuboidal epithelium, cytoplasm stains less intense and no brush border. Active reabsorption (ADH and aldosterone).

      1. Straight part—continuous with loop of Henle.
      2. Convoluted part—cortex lies close to vascular pole (JGA).

3. Medullary rays consist of straight portion of nephron and collecting tubule.

Medulla

1. Loop of Henle (descending and ascending segments). Loop of Henle as simple squamous epithelium. Descending limb (thin—15 μm)—loop of Henle, ascending limb (thin and thick—30 μm) → DCT

   Countercurrent multiplier system. Loop of Henle surrounded by vasa recta (arteries and veins).

2. Collecting ducts and papillary ducts: Collecting tubules in the cortex present in the medullary ray and also present in the medulla pyramid. It is not a part of nephron.

   It starts from DCT → end in ducts of Bellini (papillary duct). Lined by simple cuboidal epithelium with microvilli.

Functions

i. Regulation of urine formation
ii. Maintains acid–base balance
iii. Controlled by ADH
iv. Deficiency → diabetes insipidus.

Juxtaglomerular (JG) apparatus is present at vascular pole

1. TM of afferent arteriole: Smooth muscle → highly modified to form myoepithelial JG cells.
2. DCT cells modify to tall columnar → macula densa lie close to JG cells.
3. Together form JG apparatus → secrete renin → acts on angiotensinogen in blood → angiotensinogen I → enzyme in lung → angiotensinogen II → regulates BP.
4. JG cells liberate erythropoietin factor → help in maturation of RBCs.

2. Ureter: Histology

Each ureter conducts urine from the renal pelvis to the urinary bladder and is approximately 24 to 34 cm long.

Histology of ureter: Lumen is star-shape: It has three layers.

i. Mucous membrane: Inner
ii. Muscular layer: Middle
iii. Adventitia (fibrous layer): Outer.

i. **Mucous membrane is thrown into 6–8 longitudinal folds (empty)**
   1. Urothelium or transitional epithelium: 4–6 cells thickness.
      A. Deep → columnar
      B. Middle → polyhedral
      C. Surface cells → umbrella-shape with eosinophilic glycoprotein (render cells impermeable to urine)
   2. Lamina propria—wide fibroelastic connective tissue
ii. **Muscular layer**
   Smooth muscle of upper 2/3rds is thick.
      A. Inner longitudinal
      B. Outer circular (reverse GIT). Lateral 1/3rd additional outer longitudinal.
iii. **Adventitia:** Fibrous layer continuous with capsule of kidney.
   Consists of loose connective tissue (CF, EF, blood vessels, lymphatics, nerve fibers and adipocytes).

3. Urinary Bladder

A hollow organ with thick muscular wall and it is lined by transitional epithelium. The cells shapes accommodate to change depending upon on volume of urine. Mucosa of the urinary bladder with stand osmotic changes of urine. Resistant to toxic substances present in urine.

Histology of urinary bladder: Layers of similar to ureter and it is more thick.
- Mucous membrane
- Muscularis
- Serosa (superior) or adventitia (inferior lateral)
   1. Mucous membrane 6–8 cell thickness, and it is thrown into numerous folds when empty.
      a. Epithelium is transitional
         Basal cells: Cuboidal and uninucleate, diploid number of nuclei
         Middle cells: Pear shape, progressive fuse and become larger. Polyploidy nucleus.

Surface cells: Largest umbrella shape, octoploidy. Luminal surface covered glycoprotein embedded in lipid bilayer → withstands stretching and maintains osmotic pressure between urine and underlying tissue. Transitional epithelium is now also considered as pseudostratified appearance.

b. Lamina propria: Superficial, it is dense fibroelastic and deep is loose connective tissue and blood vessels.

2. **Muscularis:** Smooth muscle known as detrusor muscle forms a meshwork of three layers. Irregularly arranged, intermingled with each other. Internal and external are longitudinal and middle is thick circular.

3. Serosa on superior surface and adventitia on inferior lateral surface.

14

Endocrine System

HISTOLOGY

Glands with internal secretion (hormones) highly vascular with rich capillary plexus or sinusoids.

Along with ANS, endocrine organs control

1. Co-ordinate the metabolic activities.
2. Regulate the internal environment of the body.

Endocrine system consists of cells, tissues and organs that secrete hormones.

Hormones released into the interstitial connective tissue from which pass directly into blood or lymph circulation. These hormones reach their 'target organ' they and exert their specific effect. They act only on one organ or one type of cell or have wide spread effects.

Some organs are primarily endocrine organ, and some contain elements of both endocrine and exocrine.

The ovary and testes are both exocrine organs, 'producing' ova and spermatozoa respectively and are endocrine organs secreting hormones such as estrogen, progesterone and testosterone.

Pancreas, part of the organ is an exocrine gland the acini and part is endocrine the islets of Langerhans which secrete hormones.

Purely endocrine organs include the thyroid, parathyroid, adrenal and pituitary gland.

Basic microscopic structure

1. Cords
2. Clumps
3. Follicles

1. Hypophysis Cerebri or Pituitary Gland

Master endocrine gland, it influences peripheral glands and itself influenced by hypothalamus.

Pituitary gland or hypophysis cerebri lies in hypophysial fossa—two parts

I. Adenohypophysis

Pars distalis (P. anterior) anterior to cleft.
Pars intermedia: Posterior to cleft.
Pars tuberalis: Extension of pars distalis.
Anterior lobe: Pars distalis and pars intermedia. Adeno-hypophysis: Composed of glandular tissue.

II. Neurohypophysis

Pars nervosa: Posterior to pars intermedia infundibular stalk median eminence.

Posterior lobe: Pars nervosa and is (neurohypophysis) composed of neural tissue or neurosecretory tissue.

1. Adenohypohypysis forms 75% of hypophysis cerebri ectoderm (Rathke's pouch): Microscopic structure

a. Anterior pituitary or pars distalis

Highly vascular, branching cords of secretory epithelial cells. Separated by fenestrated sinusoids and reticular fibers.

Cells of pars distalis stain intensely:

1. Chromophils—50% brightly staining granules in their cytoplasm, which contain hormones.
2. Chromophobes—50% granules are not prominent cells are quiescent. They are also known as null cells. Degranulate phase of secretion.

3. According to affinity of specific granules which take up dyes

    i. Acidophils or alpha (α) 35%. Acidic dyes are eosin. *Two types*: **Somatotrophs:** Growth or somatotrophic hormone (stain with orange G are organophils) and **mammotrophs** (stain with Azocrine are carminophils): Prolactin.

    ii. Basophiles or beta (β) 15%. Basophilic dyes are hematoxylin. Basophils are also PAS +VE. Larger than acidophils with less numerous granules.

       Two types of basophils: Stain with aldehy defushin beta (β) basophils, e.g. thyrotrophs (TSH)—stimulates thyroid gland

       Do not stain with aldehyde fushin delta (δ) basophils, e.g.

       a. Corticotrophs (ACSH and MSH).

       b. Gonadotrophs (FSH and LH).

   iii. Chromophobes (50%) are reservoir cells and stem consists of degranulate secretory cells capable of giving rise to chromophils.

b. *Pars intermedia* 2% of hypophysis developed in man between PD and PN.

Consisting of vesicles or follicles filled with colloid and secretes MSH.

c. *Pars tuberalis*: Surrounds the infundibular stalk like collar. Consists of large blood vessels, admixed α and β cells.

2. Neurohypophysis or posterior pituitary (develops down growth—diencephalon)

- Pars nervosa

    a. It consists of cells, blood vessels and nonmyelinating nerves fibers as fibrillar processes. Nerve fibers are terminal ramifications of hypothalamo-hypophyseal tracts cell bodies are in paraventricular nucleus supraoptic nucleus of hypothalamus.

b. Terminals of nerve fibers (axon terminals) contain granules or hormones appear as basophilic masses known as Herring bodies.

c. Pituicytes are glial cell are supporting cells with oval nucleus with scanty cytoplasm.

2. Thyroid Gland

It consists two lateral lobes and an isthmus. Covered by capsule. Produces two hormones:

1. Thyroid hormone: Tyrosine.
2. Calcitonin involved calcium and phosphorus metabolism.

Effects of thyroid hormone (thyroxin)

Protein synthesis, bone growth, neuronal maturation and cell differentiation.

Microscopic Structure

1. Thyroid is highly vascular and composed of spherical follicles.
2. Follicular cells produce thyroglobulin, the precursor of thyroid hormone (thyroxin). Colloid in the lumen is of thyroglobulin. Follicles form the structural unit of thyroid gland.

    Vary in shape and size irregular with spherical lumen containing colloid (thyroglobin hormone).

    The colloid is PAS +ve, acidophilic when inactive and basophilic when active. Follicles are closely packed within the delicate network of reticular fibers. There is extensive fenestrated capillary bed between the follicles. Epithelium of thyroid follicles vary from flattened to cuboidal.

    a. Low epithelium: Simple squamous (flat) gland is hypoactive.

    b. High epithelium (simple cuboidal or simple columnar) hyperactive → thyroxine, T_3 or T_4.

3. Parafollicular 'C' cells produce calcitonin, are single or groups within the follicles between follicular cells and basement membrane or interfollicular tissue. They are rounded and larger than follicular cells.

Parathyroid glands: Gland presents on posterior part of thyroid gland. Parenchyma consists of cords of cells

Parenchyma consists of two types of cells:

1. Chief cells (light and dark) large vesicular nucleus granular cytoplasm. Between which dense capillary network. These are abundant cells (principal cells) that produce PTH parathormone.

2. Oxyphil cells (eosinophilic) appear just before puberty are large, acidophilic without secretory granules and dark nucleus unknown function. Not involved in hormonal synthesis.

3. Suprarenal or Adrenal Glands

Suprarenal means on top of the kidney. Adrenal cortex (outer), adrenal medulla (inner), each is → two endocrine glands and help with extreme situations. It consists of outer cortex derived from intermediate mesoderm (coelomic epithelium) with yellowish due to lipids. Inner medulla derived from neural crest cells and it is reddish brown.

Microscopic structure

1. Adrenal gland enclosed by thick capsule and it extends into gland as reticular fibers → contains arteries, veins, nerves and lymphatics.
   Septa from the capsule penetrate, the cortex contains arteries → entermedulla end in venous sinusoids.

Adrenal cortex: Exhibits three concentric zones

1. **Zona glomerulosa 15%** → mineral corticoids
   Germinative zone maintains cortex population secretes minerocorticoids. It forms the outer zone of the cortex. Small polyhedral cells arranged in form of rounded groups or curved columns. Cells deeply stained nucleus, cytoplasm is basophilic, a few lipid droplets (poorly developed humans).

2. **Zona fasciculata 75%** → glucocorticoids. It is the thickest zone. Cells are known as spongiocytes. Large polyhedral

cells, vesicular nucleus, cytoplasm basophilic with lipid droplets appear vacuolated or spongy. Cells arranged in radial cords of two rows with parallel fenestrated sinusoids between them.

3. **Zona reticularis 10%**—sex hormones. Cells are of branching interconnected cords (anatomizing) of rounded cells. There is shrunken nucleus, cytoplasm basophilic with few lipids. Less active zone—cortical cells die, known as graveyard.

Adrenal medulla: No boundary between cortex and medulla. It produces epinephrine and nor-epinephrine.

i. Medulla composed of clumps of cells chromaffin cells or pheochromocytes modified postganglionic sympathetic neurons that secrete catecholamine.

ii. Clumps of chromaffin cells are large ovoid, vesicular nucleus, cytoplasm with fine granules that stain with chromaffin salts → reddish brown.

iii. Scattered among medullary cells are sympathetic Gn (multipolar neurons).

iv. Extensive sinusoids.

Pathology and Applied

Pituitary Hypophysis Cerebri

a. Gigantism—too much growth hormone (GH) in childhood
b. Acromegaly—too much growth hormone in adulthood
c. Pituitary dwarfs—too little growth hormone in childhood
c. Diabetes insipidus—too much ADH

Pancreas: Diabetes mellitus (insulin)

Thyroid

a. Hyperthyroidism, commonest is Grave's disease (autoimmune)
b. Hypothyroidism: In childhood leads to cretinism. Endemic goiter from insufficient iodine in diet.

Male Genital System

Male genital consists of following pair
1. Pair of testes (in the scrotum)
2. Excretory ducts—epididymis, vas deferens
3. Accessory glands—prostate and seminal vesicle.

1. Testes
Testes present the scrotum (temperature 2–3° less than abdomen). Produces spermatozoa and testosterone.
  i. Testes enclosed by thick capsule.
      1. Tunica vaginalis
      2. Tunica albuginea
      3. Tunica vasculosa
  T. albuginea thickens and extends into each testis to form mediastinum testis as the septa into interior and it divides testis into 250 testicular lobules.
  ii. Each lobule contains 1–4 long convoluted seminiferous tubules. ST → converges to form straight tubules → anastomose to form rete testis → 10–20 efferent ductules of testes form epididymis (head).

Microscopic structure of testis seminiferous tubules:
1. Interstitial connective tissue which surrounds and binds seminiferous tubules.
2. In between seminiferous tubules is interstitial connective tissue consists of blood vessels, nerves, lymphatic and interstitial cells of Leydig.

3. Interstitial cells of Leydig (groups) that secrete hormone the testosterone. Cells are polyhedral situated within the lobules and outside the seminiferous tubules.
4. Each seminiferous tubule is lined stratified germinal epithelium—two types of major cell.
   (A) Proliferating spermatogonic germ cells, and
   (B) Nonproliferating supporting (Sertoli cells).
   Seminiferous tubules highly convoluted cut various sections. Surrounded outer fibrous connective tissue, lamina propria. Inner thin basement membrane has complex stratified germinal epithelium consisting of spermatogenic cells and Sertoli cells (sustenacular). External circular smooth muscle.
   Spermatogonia cells divide and differentiate → primary spermatocyte → divide (meiotic) to form spermatids.
5. Sertoli cells or nursing cells (blood testis barrier): A few in number placed along basement membrane at regular intervals.
   • Tall, slender and elongated, resting on basement membrane.
   • Cytoplasm exhibits faint longitudinal striations and nucleus ovoid.
   • Head of maturing spermatozoa lie in the deep recess.

2. Epididymis

Pair along the posterior border of testis. Head (10–20 efferent ductules). Body and tail consist of single highly convoluted duct (canal of epididymis) → continuous vas deferens.
1. Head—efferent ductules → irregular lumen with tall columnar ciliated cells alternating with short cuboidal cell and lumen with sperms.
2. Body and tail (smooth contour lumen) canal of epididymis with pseudostratified columnar with stereocilia.
3. Basal lamina of tubule surrounded—circular smooth muscle.
   Absorption of excessive tubular fluid and phagocytosis of defective spermatozoa and maturity, motility of sperms.

3. Vas deferens (Ductus deferens)

It develops from mesonephric duct. It is continuous with canal of epididymis (tail) → joins the duct of seminal vesicle → ejaculatory duct.

Ductus deferens, thick wall with 3 layers

1. Mucous membrane,
2. Muscular layer, and
3. Adventitia
   1. Mucous membrane shows number of longitudinal folds and stellate lumen. Mucous membrane consists of:
      a. Epithelium is pseudostratified columnar epithelium with stereocilia. Tall columnar cells with stereocilia and short basal cells (absorption)
      b. Thin lamina propria—CF and EF.
   2. Muscular layer: Thick with inner, thin longitudinal, middle thick circular and outer thin longitudinal.
   3. Adventitia: Dense irregular connective tissue—blood vessels, nerves and adipose cells emerges with surrounding tissue.

4. Prostate Gland: Accessory Gland

It surrounds the 1st part of urethra at its origin. Produces thin watery fluid, rich in citric acid and acid phosphatase.

Development

1. Glandular part—urogenital sinus as endodermal out growth
2. Fibromuscular part—splanchnopleuric mesoderm.

Coronal section

Prostatic urethra, seminalis colliculus, prostatic utriculus, ejaculatory duct and prostatic sinuses.

Microscopic structure

1. Glandular elements distributed three different zones concentrically arranged around the urethra.

i. Small mucosal glands, open directly into urethra.

ii. Surrounded by submucosal glands which open by short ducts.

iii. Main glands form the bulk of prostate gland, open into urethra by long ducts.

Surrounded by fibroblastic capsule containing smooth muscles.

2. Prostatic tissue, glandular alveoli are secretory acini as follicles. Small irregular branched tuboacinar of varying size. Glands embedded in fibromuscular strome, smooth M, CF and EF coursing in varying directions.

3. Prostatic urethra: Cresentic shape with small diverticulae along the lumen—transitional epithelium.

4. Seminal colliculus: Ridge of dense fibromuscular strome without glands protrudes into urethral lumen giving it cresentic shape.

5. Prostatic utriculus lies in seminal colliculus opens into urethra. It has a folded mucous membrane with simple columnar epithelium.

6. Ejaculatory duct penetrates prostate course along utriculus and opens into urethra.

7. Glandular acini: Vary in size, lumen large and irregular because core of connective tissue projects into lumen. Acini contain prostatic secretions. Epithelium of glandular acini—simple columnar or pseudostratified columnar with basal cells. In between are fibromuscular stoma (smooth muscles and CF).

8. Condensed prostatic secretions or concretions between (corpora amylase—amyloidal bodies) are glycoprotein **often** calcified in old individuals.

9. Ducts 12–20 drain into the urethra—prostatic sinuses.

10. Fibromuscular strome smooth muscle, connective tissue blend and course in all directions.

Functions

Produces thin watery and acidic fluid rich in acid phosphatase, amylase, protease, citric acid and prostaglandins (nutrition for sperms) prostate specific antigen (PSA). PSA increases in concentration in blood in malignancy of prostate.

Female Genital System

Human female reproductive organs

Internal—pair of ovaries, pair of fallopian tubes, uterus (body and cervix) vagina.

External—labium majora, labium minora, clitoris and mammary glands.

1. OVARY

Dull grey, 3 cm diameter. It is a female gonads responsible for producing ova and two hormones, the estrogen and progesterone. Hormones are responsible for cyclic changes in uterine endometrium.

1. Free surface covered with surface epithelium known as germinal epithelium—cuboidal later squamous. Beneath epithelium is tunica albuginea.
2. Deep to it is thick cortex forms the greater part and it enclose central medulla except at hilum.
3. Cortex follicles in various stages and corpus luteum. Primordial follicle (unilaminar), primary follicle (multilaminar), secondary follicle (with numerous cavities), graafian follicle (large antrum) and atretic follicles.
4. Corpus luteum-highly folded wall. Corpus albican, with glossy membrane.
5. Medulla: Interior with large blood vessels and chromaffin cell (androgen).

2. UTERINE TUBE

Three layers—internal is mucosa, middle is muscular and external is serosa

1. Mucosa shows mucosal folds. Lining epithelium is simple columnar ciliated—ciliated columnar cells, peg cells undifferentiated basal cells—stem cells. Show cyclic changes between various stages of menstrual cycle and regulated by ovarian hormones.
   Lamina propria: Cellular loose connective tissue rich blood vessels, with cavernous tissue.
2. Muscularis—two layers inner thick circular and outer thin longitudinal. In between abundant connective tissue.
3. Serosa—outer most is peritoneum. Mesothelium with loose connective tissue.

3. UTERUS

Wall of uterus has three layers

1. Endometrium (inner): Endometrium is important for implantation and nourishment of embryo. Endometrium has three phases.
   a. Proliferative (follicular) phase 5–14 days (2–4 mm thick) graafian follicle development.
   b. Secretory (luteal) phase 15–28 days (5–7 mm thick) corpus luteum formation.
   c. Menstrual phase—1–4 days: In case of fertilization, implantation of embryo fails → menstrual phase
2. Myometrium—fibromuscular + blood vessles, lymphatics and nerves.
3. Perimetrium—mesothelium—loose connective tissue.

Proliferative phase

Proliferative or follicular phase 5–14 days. It follows menstrual phase, stratum functionalis is shed. Corresponds to maturing follicle in ovary and it is under estrogen influence.

1. Endometrium 2–5 mm thick under the influence of estrogen and consists of two layers of stratum. Functionalis and stratum basalis.
2. Uterine glands are straight and coiled in basal part.
3. Blood vessels in stratum functionalis are veins and capillaries. In stratum basalis highly spiral arteries.
4. Endometrial stroma is highly cellular and fibrous.

Secretive phase

The secretory (luteal) phase 14–24 days. It starts after ovulation and corresponds to development of corpus luteum. It is under the influence of progesterone and estrogen.

1. Endometrium 5–7 mm thick under the influence of both progesterone and estrogen stratum functionalis consists of two layers, i.e. stratum compactum + stratum spongiosum and stratum basalis.
2. Uterine glands are corkscrew shape and rich in secretions
3. Blood vessels: In stratum functionalis veins and capillaries with coiled arteries in stratum basalis.
4. Endometrial stroma highly cellular and edematous.

Menstrual phase 1–4 days

1. Starts when fertilization and implantation fails to occur.
2. Fall of progesterone and oestrogen levels in blood due to regression of corpus luteum.
3. Endometrium loses its epithelium and much of underlying tissues.
4. Eroded surface covered with blood clots, fragments of endometrium and uterine glands.
5. Superficial part of uterine glands filled with blood. Fundi (deep) of uterine glands intact.
6. Stratum functionalis—RBCs, infiltration of WBCs and lymphocyte.

Menstruation: Vaginal discharge. It consists of fragments of stroma, blood clots, uterine glands and cells.

4.MAMMARY GLAND

A mammary gland is an apocrine gland. In female that produces milk to feed young offspring. The mammary glands are modified sweat glands located in subcutaneous tissue of pectoral region. Present in both sexes.

In the inactive mammary gland

1. Glandular elements consist only of ducts.
2. The intralobular ducts and terminal interlobular ducts are lined with simple cuboidal, epithelium, supported by basement membrane.
3. Myoepithelial cells lies between the intralobular duct cells and the basement membrane.
4. Within the lobules, that surrounds the intralobular ducts is loose and highly vascular. It contains a large number of cells such as fibroblasts, lymphocytes and plasma cells and little fat.
5. The lobules are separated from one another by dense connective tissue that may contain abundant adipose tissue.

Mammary gland during pregnancy

1. The ducts in the lobules proliferate and branch and secretory alveoli sprout from them.
2. Alveoli are spherical cuboidal epithelial and become active milk—secreting structures. Myoepithelial cells at present their base.
3. Alveoli difficult distinguish from ducts.
4. Increase in glandular tissue is accompanied by a decrease in the connective and adipose tissue.
5. Lobules are separated reduced strands of dense interlobular connective tissue with plasma cells and lymphocytes.

5. PLACENTA

1. Foetal part is chorionic plate (trophoblast and connective tissue) and anchoring villi arising from it and with floating villi in intervillous spaces.

2. Maternal part is decidua basalis it is functional layer of endometrium.

3. Deep basal layer is basal part of glands and spiral arteries.

4. Myometrium.

Central Nervous System

1. HISTOLOGY OF SPINAL CORD

Spinal cord or spinal medulla above continuous medulla oblongata, below end at conus medullaris occupies upper 2/3rds of vertebral column.

1. Transverse section of spinal cord: Inner grey matter (H-shaped) outer white matter.

2. Grey matter: Neurons cell bodies, dendrites and axon (non-myelinated), neuroglia cells, blood vessels arranged in H-shaped fluted column.

3. White matter: Myelinated nerve fibers (axons), neuroglia cells and blood vessels. It occupies outside the butterfly-shaped central grey matter.

4. Each half of spinal cord the grey matter is divisible: Large ventral mass → anterior (ventral) grey column (horn) and narrow elongated posterior or dorsal grey column (horn).

5. Thoracic region → small lateral projection of grey → lateral grey column (horn).

6. White matter of spinal cord is divided into right and left halves in front by deep anterior median fissure and behind by posterior median sulcus and septum.

7. White matter contains ascending and descending tracts that connect grey matter at different levels of spinal cord, brainstem, cerebellum or cerebral cortex.

2. CEREBELLUM IS PART OF HINDBRAIN

Head ganglion of proprioceptive system and maintain equilibrium and posture of body.

Cerebellum consists of median vermis and two large lateral hemispheres.

Functional or physiological classification

i. Vestibular cerebellum (archicerebellum)
ii. Spinocerebellum (paleocerebellum)
iii. Cerebrocerebellum (neocerebellum)

1. Cerebellum has outer grey matter known as cerebellar cortex and inner white matter is medullary core (arbor vitae).
2. Deep intracerebellar nuclei (4 pairs): Dentate nucleus, interpositus nucleus, fastigii nucleus which are present in the white matter.

Histology of Cerebellar Cortex—Three Layers

Uniform structure seen in all parts of cerebellum.

1. Outer molecular layer: A few cells and horizontal nerve fibers. Two types of neurons—stellate and basket cells. Nerve fibers are parallel.
2. Middle Purkinje cell layer: Piriform or large flask shaped cells forming a single stratum of cells. Dendrites ramiphy into molecular layer. Axons arise bottom of cell body and extend into granular layer → white matter and end in deep cerebellar nuclei.
3. Inner granular layer which rest on white matter → core of cerebellar folium consists of myelinated axons. Granular cells dark staining with little cytoplasm. Golgi cells large with vesicular nucleus and more cytoplasm. Throughout are clear spaces called glomeruli (synaptic complexes).

White matter → core of cerebellar folium consists of myelinated axons which are afferents (S, M and I) or sensory inputs of cerebellum (climbing fibers and mossy fibers) efferents → peduncles (S and I).

3. CEREBRAL CORTEX

Cerebral hemisphere has outer grey matter → cerebral cortex or pallium and inner white matter. Subcortical nuclei in the white core → basal ganglia subdivision of cerebral cortex.

1. Allocortex: Archicortex (archipallium) and palaeocortex (paleopallium).
2. Isocortex: Neocortex (neopallium).

Neocortex or neopallium is 90% of cortex. Made up of six superimposed lamina.

Different types of cell are distributed in six layers, with one or more cell types predominant in each layer. Horizontal and radial axons associated neuronal cells in different layers give laminated appearance.

   i. Plexiform (molecular): Dendrites and axons of cortical neurons making synapses; neuroglia and horizontal cells.
  ii. Outer granular cell: Dense population small stellate cells [small neurons] and a few pyramidal cells; various axons and dendrites connections.
 iii. Outer pyramidal cell: Moderate size; increasing size deeper lamina.
 iv. Inner granular: Densely packed stellate cells.
  v. Ganglionic or inner pyramidal: Large pyramidal cells (Betz cells) and a few stellate cells.
 vi. Multiform cell: Numerous small neurons, small pyramidal cells, stellate cells and Martinotti cells superficially and fusiform cells in deeper part.

18

Special Senses

1. Lacrimal Gland: Two Parts (Orbital and Palpebral)

Secretes tears and its ducts convey the fluid into conjunctival sac.

1. Lacrimal gland consists of several lobes, divided into fine lobules by connective septa.
   That contain nerves, blood vessels and adipose tissue.
2. Secretory portions are serous acini with myoepithelial cells. Gland divided into lobes by connective tissue. Columnar secretory cells have pale granules and secrete Antibacterial lysozyme.
3. Two types of cells (EM): K cells(mucus) and G cells (serous), possibly represent different stages of secretory activity of cells. Secretions are alkaline (enzymes and lysozyme bactericidal) 1 ml/per day.
4. Acini of vary size and shape lined by simple columnar epithelium resting on basement membrane. Myoepithelial cells surround the alveoli.
5. Secretory motor nerve is facial nerve (parasympathetic).

2. Cornea: Outer Tunic

It forms anterior 1/6th of the eyeball.

Thick, avascular and transparent, projecting with convex anteriorly. It is site of light entering. Microscopically cornea has five layers.

1. Corneal epithelium continuous with conjunctival epithelium. It covers the anterior surface of cornea. Nonpapillated, nonkeratinized stratified squamous epithelium (5th cell thick).

2. Anterior limiting lamina or Bowman's membrane. Acellular and made up of fine CF embedded in the matrix.

3. Substantia propria or corneal stroma forms the bulk and thickest part of cornea. Compact and transparent, made up of 200–250 lamella of parallel type I CF with fibroblast (keratocytes/corneal corpuscles) embedded in ground substance. Macrophages, lymphocytes and neutrophils+

4. Posterior limiting lamina or Descemet's membrane: Acellular, thin homogenous, collagenous layer regarded as basement membrane of posterior corneal epithelium which the endothelium.

5. Endothelium covers the posterior surface of cornea. It is simple cuboidal epithelium which constitutes the endothelium of anterior chamber. It is in contact with aqueous humor and also line iridocorneal angle.

3. Retina: Neural Tunic of the Eyeball

It derived from two layers

Of invaginated optic cup, from forebrain. Outer layer is pigment cell layer; inner layer is complex multilaminar. Anterior to ora serrata the retina is two layers (non nervous stratum). Posterior 2/3rds is retina proper: 10 layers → contain variety of cell types.

Choroid → vitreous humor, the retina consists of 10 layers

1. Pigment cell layer: Outermost layer of retina. Simple cuboidal cells with microvilli and melanin granules in cytoplasm and their processes extend between rods and cones. *Function*: Absorption of excessive light and prevents reflexion. Mechanical support rods and cones.

2. *Layer of rods and cones* is photoreceptors. It consists of outer and inner segment of rods and cones of peripheral processes. Rods are slender and cones are thick.

3. *Outer limiting membrane* (OLM) formed by processes of neuroglia cells, the Müller cells (fusiform).

4. *Outer nuclear layer* contains several layers cell bodies and nuclei of rods and cones with scanty cytoplasm forming thin rim. Rods and cones are modified neuron.

   i. Peripheral process (outer segment) and inner segment contains large number of mitochondria.

   ii. Cell body with nuclei (ONL)

   iii. Inner process: Axon of rod spherule and cone pedicle form synapse with bipolar cells (OPL).

5. *Outer plexiform layer* complexes synaptic interaction between axons of rods and cones with dendrites of bipolar neurons (INL) and also with processes of horizontal cells.

6. *Inner nuclear layer* contains bipolar cells and associated neurons, the horizontal cells, amacrine cell and neuroglia, Müller cells nuclei (INL).

7. *Inner plexiform layer*

   1. Axons of bipolar neurons synapse with dendrites of ganglionic cells (GCL).

   2. Axons of bipolar cells with amacrine process.

8. *Ganglionic cell layer* consists of cell bodies of ganglionic cells and neuroglia cells (Müller) its dendrites with axon of bipolar cells. Its axons form the optic nerve (non-myelinated) which converge towards optic disc. Two types of ganglionic cells → monosynaptic and polysynaptic.

9. *Optic nerve layer*: Non-myelinated axons of ganglionic cells. Fibers converge to optic disc → pass through lamina cibrose sclera → optic nerve (myelinated axons of ganglionic cells form the nerve fibers and the optic nerve.

10. *Inner limiting membrane*: Separates retina from vitreous body and supports, provide nutrition to retina. The terminations of inner fibers of Müller cells (retinal glial) which expand to form the tenth layer (ILM).

Photosensitive retina contains three types of neurons distributed in 3 layers—rods and cones (2, 4 layer), bipolar cells (6-INL) and ganglionic cells (8 layer).

INTERNAL EAR

Function is hearing and equilibrium. It consists of labyrinth means complexity of its shape. Internal ear consists of bony labyrinth and membranous labyrinth which lie in with in the petrous temporal bone.

Osseous labyrinth—18 mm long; consists of series of bony spaces lined internally by periosteum filled with perilymph which is similar to extracellular fluid. There are cochlea, vestibule and three semicircular canals.

Membranous labyrinth consists of series of membranous sacs and tubes contained within bony labyrinth filled with endolymph similar to intracellular fluid. There are cochlear duct, utricle and saccule and three semicircular ducts.

Cochlear duct–Scala media-2 $\frac{3}{4}$ th turns begins at copula the lagena, basal turn enters vestibule and joins ductus reuniens and continuous saccule. Organ of Corti, the peripheral organ of hearing lies on cochlear duct.

Organ of Corti rests on basilar membrane with no blood vessel and nourished by Corti lymph. It consists of:

1. Inner rod (6000) and outer rod cells (4000) (pillar on) basilar membrane enclosing tunnel of Corti (Corti lymph).
2. Inner hair (3500) and outer hair cells (12000–20000) sensory cells and are the innervated by cochlear nerve. Apex microvilli (stereocilia). Tectorial membrane cellular protein covers stereocilia hair cells.
3. Supporting cells (phalangeal or deiters, Hensen and claudius).

Applied Histology

- Tinnitus: Ringing noise, deafness—peripheral cochlear disease.
- Vertigo: Giddiness—labyrinthine dysfunction associated with nystagmus.
- Motion sickness: Vertigo, headache and vomiting—excess stimulation of saccular and utricle (deaf and mute—no receptors—no motion sickness).
- Meniere's disease: Paroxysmal attacks of vertigo, tinnitus and progressive hearing loss.
- Cerebellopontine tumors involve 7 and 8 cranial nerves.